Emergencies in Respiratory Medicine

Published and forthcoming titles in the Emergencies in . . . series:

Emergencies in Paediatrics and Neonatology
Stuart Crisp

Emergencies in Adult Nursing
Edited by Philip Downing

Emergencies in Anaesthesia
Edited by Keith Allman, Andrew McIndoe, and Iain H. Wilson

Emergencies in Children's and Young People's Nursing
Edited by E.A. Glasper, Gill McEwing, and Jim Richardson

Emergencies in Clinical Surgery
Edited by Chris Callaghan, Chris Watson and Andrew Bradley

Emergencies in Critical Care, 2e
Edited by Martin Beed, Richard Sherman, and Ravi Mahajan

Emergencies in Gastroenterology and Hepatology
Marcus Harbord and Daniel Marks

Emergencies in Mental Health Nursing
Edited by Patrick Callaghan

Emergencies in Obstetrics and Gynaecology
Edited by S. Arulkumaran

Emergencies in Oncology
Edited by Martin Scott-Brown, Roy A.J. Spence, and Patrick G. Johnston

Emergencies in Paediatrics and Neonatology, 2e
Edited by Stuart Crisp and Jo Rainbow

Emergencies in Palliative and Supportive Care
Edited by David Currow and Katherine Clark

Emergencies in Primary Care
Chantal Simon, Karen O'Reilly, John Buckmaster, and Robin Proctor

Emergencies in Psychiatry, 2e
Basant Puri and Ian Treasaden

Emergencies in Respiratory Medicine
Edited by Robert Parker, Catherine Thomas, and Lesley Bennett

Emergencies in Sports Medicine
Edited by Julian Redhead and Jonathan Gordon

Head, Neck and Dental Emergencies
Edited by Mike Perry

Medical Emergencies in Dentistry
Nigel Robb and Jason Leitch

Emergencies in Respiratory Medicine

SECOND EDITION

EDITED BY

Ryan Robinson

Specialty Trainee in Respiratory Medicine and General Internal Medicine, Wirral University Teaching Hospital, Wirral, UK

Ruth Cade

Specialty Trainee in Respiratory and General Internal Medicine, Mersey and West Lancashire Teaching Hospitals Trust, Prescot, UK

OXFORD
UNIVERSITY PRESS

OXFORD
UNIVERSITY PRESS

Great Clarendon Street, Oxford, OX2 6DP,
United Kingdom

Oxford University Press is a department of the University of Oxford. It furthers the University's objective of excellence in research, scholarship, and education by publishing worldwide. Oxford is a registered trade mark of Oxford University Press in the UK and in certain other countries.

First Edition published in 2007
Second Edition published in 2026

Published in the United States of America by Oxford University Press
198 Madison Avenue, New York, NY 10016, United States of America.

British Library Cataloguing in Publication Data
Data available

Library of Congress Control Number: 2026931248

ISBN 978–0–19–891833–2

DOI: 10.1093/med/9780198918332.001.0001

Printed in India by
Replika Press Pvt. Ltd.

FSC
www.fsc.org
MIX
Paper | Supporting responsible forestry
FSC™ C016779

Preface

Anyone involved in the care of Respiratory patients will be faced with emergency situations at some point. This book aims to equip the reader with a concise and practical approach to their assessment and management, when the need arises.

The book is divided into five sections. The first covers common acute respiratory presentations. The second covers particular acute clinical presentations. The third section covers specific problems seen in a range of common chronic respiratory conditions. The final two sections cover practical management issues and key investigations.

It has been an honour to update the latest version of this title, the first of which was edited by Robert Parker, Catherine Thomas and Lesley Bennett. We are indebted to the original contributors (Matt Brookes, Ali Gates, James Hull, Christopher Loew, Robert MacKenzie Ross, Anjani Prasad, Najib Rahman, Fran Sinfield, Andrew Stanton, Sam Waddy and David Waine) for their succinct and insightful chapters which have been a delight to update, where needed. Much has changed in Respiratory medicine since the original edition was published in 2007, but the fundamentals remain the same.

Preface

Contents

Contributors

Renu Abraham
Respiratory Physiotherapist, Liverpool University Hospitals Foundation Trust, Liverpool, UK

Laurence Allan
Specialty Trainee in Intensive Care Medicine, Liverpool University Hospitals Foundation Trust, Liverpool, UK

Annemarie Brunswicker
Specialty Trainee in Cardiothoracic Surgery, Liverpool Heart and Chest Hospital, Liverpool, UK

Ruth Cade
Specialty Trainee in Respiratory and General Internal Medicine, Mersey and West Lancashire Teaching Hospitals Trust, Prescot, UK

Ffion Carlin
Acute Medicine Consultant, Salford Royal Hospital, Northern Care Alliance, Greater Manchester, UK

Freddy Frost
Specialty Trainee in Respiratory Medicine and General Internal Medicine, Liverpool Heart and Chest Hospital, Liverpool, UK

David Green
Specialty Trainee in Respiratory Medicine and General Internal Medicine, Liverpool Heart and Chest Hospital, Liverpool, UK

Ayesha Kumar
Consultant in Respiratory and General Internal Medicine, Liverpool University Hospitals Foundation Trust, Liverpool, UK

Kostas Liatsikos
Specialty Trainee in Respiratory Medicine and General Internal Medicine, Wirral University Teaching Hospital, Wirral, UK

Arafat Mulla
Consultant in Respiratory and General Internal Medicine, University Hospital Monklands, Lanarkshire, UK

Rebecca Nightingale
Clinical lecturer,
Centre for Tuberculosis and Department of Clinical Sciences, Liverpool School of Tropical Medicine, Liverpool, UK

Honorary consultant respiratory physiotherapist,
Department of Respiratory Medicine, Liverpool University Hospitals Foundation Trust,
Liverpool, UK

Vicki Randles
Specialty Trainee in Respiratory Medicine and General Internal Medicine, Liverpool University Hospitals Foundation Trust, Liverpool, UK

Ryan Robinson
Specialty Trainee in Respiratory Medicine and General Internal Medicine, Wirral University Teaching Hospital, Wirral, UK

Rebecca J Shaw
Specialty Trainee in Haematology, Liverpool University Hospitals Foundation Trust, Liverpool, UK

Emergency symbols

A true life-threatening emergency. Memorising these conditions may help. Call immediately for help. Try to remain calm and quickly assess ABC. Once the problem has been dealt with remember to reassess—other problems may have been forgotten or missed in the heat of the moment.

These people need to be assessed very quickly, because they can rapidly deteriorate. Consider senior help/advice as you assess the person.

These conditions require careful assessment and correction but are unlikely to become life-threatening emergencies.

These sections cover management guidelines or advice on clinical dilemmas. The timing of clinical intervention is under the control of you, their caring clinician.

Abbreviations

ABGs	arterial blood gases
ABPA	allergic bronchopulmonary aspergillosis
ACTs	airway clearance techniques
AFS	acid-fast bacilli
AMS	acute mountain sickness
Anti-GBM	anti-glomerular basement membrane
ARDS	acute respiratory distress syndrome
ARVs	anti-retrovirals
BPD	breathing pattern disorder
CAP	community-acquired pneumonia
CF	cystic fibrosis
CICO	can't intubate, can't oxygenate
CMV	cytomegalovirus
COP	cryptogenic organising pneumonia
COPD	chronic obstructive pulmonary disease
FBC	full blood count
EBUS-TBNA	endobronchial ultrasound-guided transbronchial needle aspiration
eFONA	emergency front of neck access
GPA	granulomatosis with polyangiitis
HACE	high-altitude cerebral oedema
HAPE	high-altitude pulmonary oedema
HCT	haematocrit
HFNO	high-flow nasal oxygen
HFOV	high frequency oscillatory ventilation
ILO	inducible laryngeal obstruction
IPF	idiopathic pulmonary fibrosis
IRIS	immune-reconstitution inflammatory syndrome
LTOT	long-term oxygen therapy
MC&S	microscopy, culture, and sensitivities
NIV	non-invasive ventilation
NSAIDs	nonsteroidal anti-inflammatory drugs
OIs	opportunistic infections
OSA	obstructive sleep apnoea
PA	posteroanterior
PCA	patient-controlled analgesia
PE	pulmonary embolism
PEEP	positive end-expiratory pressure
PEFR	peak expiratory flow rate
PID	pelvic inflammatory disease
PJP	Pneumocystis jiroveci pneumonia
PND	paroxysmal nocturnal dyspnoea
PT	respiratory physiotherapy
QoL	quality of life
SGAD	supraglottic airway device
SOB	shortness of breath
SVCO	superior vena cava obstruction
TENS	transcutaneous electrical nerve stimulation
TFTs	thyroid function tests
VTE	venous thromboembolism

Part 1

Presentations

Chapter 1

The peri-arrest patient

Basic life support

Occasionally you will be the first person on the scene. Doctors get used to running arrests, so do not freeze when you walk into a cubicle and find the unresponsive patient—just do the basics.

These algorithms are included as a reminder of previously learnt basic and advanced life support skills as taught on the appropriate resuscitation council courses. For further information and reading: www.resus.org.uk

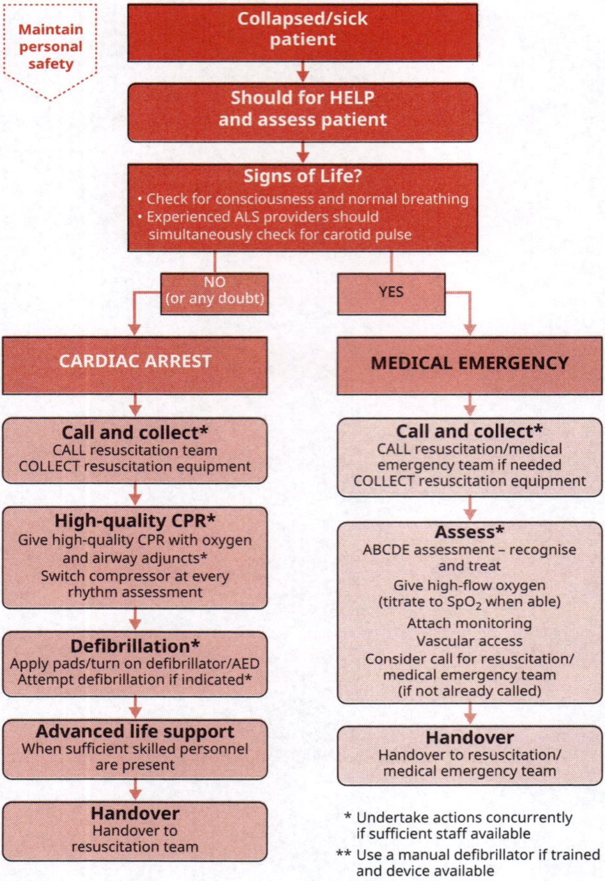

Fig. 1.1 Current basic life support algorithm. Reproduced with kind permission from the Resuscitation Council.

Advanced life support

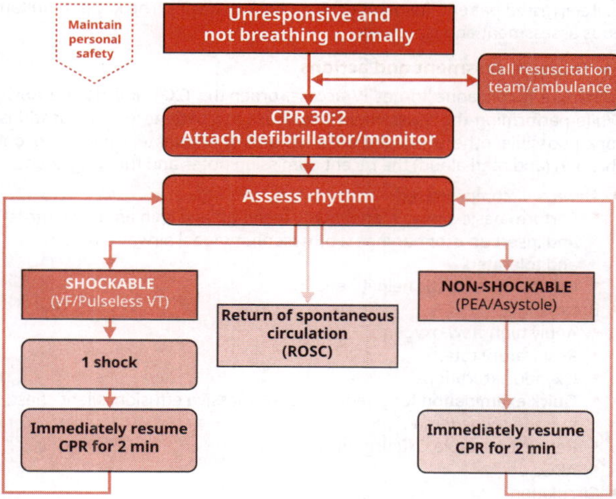

Give high-quality chest compressions, and:
- Give oxygen
- Use waveform capnography
- Continuous compressions if advanced airway
- Minimise interruptions to compressions
- Intravenous or intraosseous access
- Give adrenaline every 3–5 min
- Give amiodarone after 3 shocks
- Identify and treat reversible causes

Identify and treat reversible causes
- Hypoxia
- Hypovolaemia
- Hypo-/hyperkalaemia/ metabolic
- Hypo/hyperthermia
- Thrombosis – coronary or pulmonary
- Tension pneumothorax
- Tamponade – cardiac
- Toxins

Consider ultrasound imaging to identify reversible causes

Consider
- Coronary angiography/ percutaneous coronary intervention
- Mechanical chest compressions to facilitate transfer/ treatment
- Extracorporeal CPR

After ROSC
- Use an ABCDE approach
- Aim for SpO_2 of 94–98% and normal $PaCO_2$
- 12-lead ECG
- Identify and treat cause
- Temperature control

Fig. 1.2 Current advanced life support algorithm. Reproduced with kind permission from the Resuscitation Council.

The peri-arrest patient

Junior doctors are frequently paralysed when faced with a nearly but not quite arrested patient. Remember to go back to basics. The key is simultaneous assessment and treatment.

▶▶ Initial assessment and actions

Nominate a colleague to get IV access, order the CXR, and do the ABGs. While performing the assessment below ask the patient for a focused history if possible; otherwise ask the nurses and/or nominate someone to look through (and read aloud) the recent admission notes and the drug chart.

- Airway—if compromised
  - Perform basic airway manoeuvres (head tilt and chin lift or jaw thrust) and insert an oropharyngeal or nasopharyngeal airway if required and tolerated.
  - Call for anaesthetic help if needed.
- Breathing
  - Apply high-flow oxygen.
  - Respiratory rate.
  - Oxygen saturations.
  - Quick examination for pneumothorax, massive effusion, silent chest, pulmonary oedema.
  - Request portable CXR urgently.
  - ABGs.
- Circulation
  - Heart rate, rhythm.
  - Blood pressure.
  - JVP.
  - Capillary refill time.
  - Quick palpation of the abdomen (distended? pulsatile mass?)
  - Insert large-bore IV cannula and send FBC, U&E, Clotting ± group and save.
  - 12 lead ECG.
  - 250–500 ml fluid bolus unless heart failure/intrinsic cardiogenic shock.
- Disability
  - Capillary blood glucose.
  - AVPU assessment (Alert, responds to Voice, Pain, Unresponsive).
  - Pupils.
  - Neck stiffness.
  - Tone, plantars.

Diagnosis and treatment

The differential diagnosis of a collapsed patient is wide. At this stage you need to decide what the priority treatment is and act. Many patients will have combinations of the causes listed, e.g. a patient recently returned to the ward from intensive care may have critical care neuromyopathy and a hospital-acquired pneumonia, both causing compromise, and then become 'tipped over' by accumulation of opiate analgesia.

Airway Compromise

▶ Call for early anaesthetic help.

- Most commonly due to decreased level of consciousness. Consider:
  - ❗ **Opiates** (give naloxone 400 mcg IV stat up to 2 mg repeated at intervals of 2–3 min to a maximum of 10 mg). Remember that the half-life of naloxone is short and that half-time of opiates can be very prolonged in the critically ill. Always check for the presence of long-acting opiate patches and remove.
  - **Glucose** (if low give 50 ml 5% glucose IV stat). Diabetic patients may be symptomatically hypoglycaemic at higher levels, treat if <4.0.
  - **Intracerebral event:** bleed, coning, infection. Urgent CT head.
- Primary airway pathology:
  - **Anaphylaxis** and **anaphylactoid reactions** (➔ Chapter 18). Give IM adrenaline 0.5 mg into anterolateral thigh. Give IV fluids. Repeat IM adrenaline after 5 minutes if problems persist.
    Consider a non-sedating antihistamine when stabilised.
  - **Infection:** epiglottitis, diphtheria, uvula infection/inflammation.
  - Uncommonly, inhaled foreign body (➔ Chapter 11).

Breathing

Think through the respiratory pathway:

- **Central drive:** see opiates above; major intracerebral events, subclinical status epilepticus.
- **Nerve transmission:** high spinal cord lesion usually due to trauma (consider this in the elderly rheumatoid patient who falls on the ward—immobilise the neck). Guillain–Barré syndrome.
- **Neuromuscular:** myasthenia, Eaton–Lambert, occasionally in the immediately post-operative patient with insufficient reversal.
- **Muscular:** some will be obvious, such as Duchenne's muscular dystrophy, but beware post-ICU patients.
- **Pulmonary**: most common:
  - Infection: if appropriate these patients are likely to need respiratory support.
  - Bronchospasm: section on Asthma (➔ Chapter 20).
  - Pneumothorax: algorithm (➔ Chapter 27).

Circulation

- **Non-cardiogenic:**
  - Hypovolaemia.
  - Sepsis and vasodilatation.
  - Anaphylaxis.
  - Vasodilatory drugs.
- **Cardiogenic:**
  - Intrinsic: ischaemia, valves, arrhythmia, failure.
  - Extrinsic: pulmonary embolus, cardiac tamponade, tension pneumothorax.

Immediate actions

Airway

- Airway not compromised: continue below.

- Airway compromised: use simple manoeuvres, insert an oropharyngeal or nasopharyngeal airway.
- Remove foreign bodies if possible and visible, but remember good-fitting dentures may assist with maintaining an airway.
- Ensure suction is available, and switched on.
- Nominate an appropriate person to look after the airway; call for anaesthetic help if appropriate (see below).

Breathing

- Apply high-flow oxygen (see opposite for discussion of chronic CO_2 retention and the peri-arrest patient).
- If signs of tension pneumothorax perform needle decompression, second intercostal space, mid-clavicular line; use an IV cannula at least 18G (➔ Chapter 27).
- If evidence of bronchospasm apply continuous beta-2 agonist nebulisers driven with oxygen.
- If conscious level is preserved but hypoxic or with pulmonary oedema consider early use of CPAP (➔ Chapter 44).
- Consider whether NIV is appropriate (COPD exacerbation, hypercapnia, pH < 7.35; ➔ Chapter 8).

⚠ Do not attempt to intubate a patient yourself who is not in cardio-respiratory arrest.

Call an anaesthetist (or ICU) if:

- Severe respiratory failure.
- RR <10 or >30.
- PaO_2 <10 on high-flow oxygen.
- Rising $PaCO_2$ and acidosis.
- Decreased conscious level (AVPU P or U).
- Airway compromise, anatomical or oedema.
- Cardioversion needed and patient conscious (! if your patient is severely compromised, e.g. hypotensive in VT with impaired conscious level and needs cardioversion, do not delay. Give 2–5 mg midazolam IV, increased if necessary in steps of 1 mg to a maximum of 7.5 mg, and cardiovert).

Circulation

- Get good IV access. Consider intraosseous access in an emergency where vascular access is difficult or likely to be delayed.
- If symptomatic bradycardia give IV atropine 500 mcg, repeat as necessary to 3 mg and consider isoprenaline infusion (5 mcg min^{-1} starting dose) or external pacing.
- Provided patient is not in heart failure and does not have intrinsic cardiogenic shock then give fluid challenge (250 ml or 500 ml crystalloid) and repeat if beneficial and required.
- If the patient remains hypotensive then obtain central access and fill to a CVP of 8–12 cm. Vasoactive drugs may then be required.

● Hypercapnia and the peri-arrest patient

The majority of hypercapnic peri-arrest patients require high-flow oxygen; therefore if no medical information is available this treatment should be started. If the patient is known to have COPD with chronic hypoxia and chronic hypercapnia, titrate the O_2 concentration to the level required to achieve an SaO_2 of 88–92% using venturi adaptors.

If the patient remains hypoxic, hypercapnic, and acidotic then they will need respiratory support (either NIV or intubation and ventilation).

Further circulatory management

►► If your patient is extremely hypotensive (systolic <70 mmHg) while you are setting up your central access kit you may need to give very small boluses of peripheral vasopressors. Adrenaline is always available as 1:10 000 minijets (1 mg in 10 ml) on the arrest trolley and 0.5–1.0 ml (50–100 mcg) boluses can be given every 3–5 minutes to maintain a blood pressure. This can also be used in refractory bradycardia whilst setting up external pacing or obtaining equipment.

Vasoactive drugs are used to maintain a sensible perfusion pressure and hopefully cardiac output. Expertise is needed in using these and at this stage you should have the intensive care team to help. The following is provided as a reminder.

❗ Must be via central line unless stated otherwise. Patients should have ECG monitoring continuously and invasive arterial pressure monitoring established as soon as possible: set non-invasive BP cuff to record every 3–5 minutes in the interim. Starting doses are assuming a 70 kg adult.

Vasoconstrictors

Noradrenaline

- Pure vasoconstriction (at usual doses) so will increase BP with little effect on cardiac output.
- Usually given as 40 mcg/ml 0.9% saline; start at 10–20 ml/hour and titrate upwards.

Metaraminol

- Pure vasoconstrictor. Slower onset and offset than noradrenaline so can be given in small boluses peripherally.
- Usually dilute 10 mg (1 ml ampoule) in 20 ml 0.9% saline and given in 1–2 ml aliquots.
- Often used to maintain BP at time of induction and intubation in sick patients.

Inoconstrictors: increase blood pressure and cardiac output

Adrenaline

- As an infusion 5 ml of 1:10 000 at a rate of 1 ml (100 mcg)/minute.
- In extremis (see above) 10 ml from 1:10 000 minijet (1 mg).

Ephedrine

❗ Do not confuse with adrenaline (see above).

- Slower onset and longer lasting than adrenaline and much less potent.
- Usually dilute 30 mg (1 ml ampoule) in 10 ml 0.9% saline and give as bolus of 3 mg (1 ml).
- Often used at induction/intubation to maintain BP.

Inodilators

Dobutamine

- Will increase cardiac output and vasodilate, thereby offloading the myocardium and increasing peripheral perfusion. In some circumstances (underfilled, misdiagnosed sepsis) this will result in a dramatic fall in BP. Will increase both heart rate and contractility.
- Dilute to 0.5–1 mg/ml in 0.9% saline and infuse at 2.5–10 mcg/kg/minute.
- Often used (in conjunction with a constrictor such as noradrenaline) to improve tissue perfusion, as inferred from central venous oxygen saturations (see below).

Vasodilators

GTN

- Used to treat refractory angina or LVF.
- Boluses given sublingually (usually 500 μg).
- As an infusion 100–400 mcg/ml in 0.9% saline and infuse at 10–200 mcg/minute if required. Tolerance develops over 24–48 hours of continuous infusion.

Ongoing management

Ideally by this stage the patient is becoming stable and you have worked out the cause of the deterioration and initiated appropriate treatment. You should have the results of capillary glucose, CXR, ABG, and 12-lead ECG, and formal bloods should be on their way. If the diagnosis remains elusive, try to obtain an emergency echocardiogram. This will tell you:

- Regional wall motion abnormalities which may suggest ischaemia.
- May inform you about pulmonary artery pressures and RV function.
- Will occasionally show direct evidence of pulmonary embolism such as thrombus in transit.

This patient is clearly sick and likely to benefit from level 2 or 3 care, which will involve liaison with the Intensive Care team.

⚠ Do not attempt to transfer the patient to the CT scanner or high dependency unit without achieving stability, ensuring adequate monitoring and having appropriately trained staff. Again this will often involve liaison with the ICU team.

Targets

Normality is often difficult to achieve so what is reasonable in the short term when stabilising the peri-arrest patient? The following are a guide.

- RR <25.
- SaO_2 >90% (lower if COPD).
- HR 60–100 (accept outside this if other parameters acceptable).

- Mean arterial pressure >65 mmHg (higher if chronic hypertension).
- CVP 8–12 (or >3 cm above baseline pre-resuscitation and sustained).
- Capillary refill time <2 seconds.
- Urine output >0.5 ml/kg/hour.
- Normal conscious level.
- Arterial pH >7.25.
- Lactate <2.0 mmol/L (higher suggests poor perfusion).
- Central venous oxygen saturation ($ScvO_2$) >70%.

Driving targets beyond this is unlikely to give incremental benefit.

Chapter 2

Dyspnoea

Dyspnoea

The American Thoracic Society defines dyspnoea as 'a term used to characterize a subjective experience of breathing discomfort that is comprised of qualitatively distinct sensations that vary in intensity. The experience derives from interactions among multiple physiological, psychological, social and environmental factors and may include secondary physiological and behavioural responses.'

Dyspnoea is a common symptom and the presenting complaint of the majority of patients with respiratory disease. Acute dyspnoea usually comes on over the course of minutes to hours. Associated symptoms and signs may help with clues to the aetiology. Chronic dyspnoea occurs in the majority of respiratory conditions, the commonest being COPD and interstitial lung disease, as well as a number of cardiac conditions.

In many respiratory conditions causing chronic dyspnoea, patients will present with acute on chronic dyspnoea due to an exacerbation of their underlying condition, superimposed infection, a complication of their existing disease, such as pneumothorax or PE, or unrelated pathology.

Many causes of dyspnoea present with a normal CXR and this should not rule out a respiratory cause.

Causes of acute dyspnoea

Respiratory

- Acute asthma exacerbation.
- Exacerbation of COPD (often occurs on a background of chronic dyspnoea).
- Pneumonia.
- Pneumothorax.
- Pulmonary embolus.
- Acute hypersensitivity pneumonitis.
- Hyperventilation: need to exclude underlying cause.

Cardiovascular

- Pulmonary oedema.
- Arrhythmia.
- Cardiac tamponade.

Other

- Anaphylaxis.
- Metabolic acidosis.
- Salicylate overdose.

Causes of subacute dyspnoea

Recent onset dyspnoea (days, weeks) may precede admission to hospital. This makes new sub-acute conditions more likely and includes those listed above plus the following.

Respiratory

- Pleural effusion.
- Lung malignancy.

- Exacerbation of bronchiectasis/cystic fibrosis.
- Cryptogenic organising pneumonia.
- Acute interstitial pneumonia.
- Pulmonary vasculitis.
- Lymphangitis carcinomatosis.

Cardiovascular

- Congestive cardiac failure.
- Myocarditis.
- SVCO.

Other

- Anaemia.
- Thyrotoxicosis.

Causes of chronic dyspnoea

Chronic dyspnoea may be the presenting feature to the emergency department, but more usually presents as an acute worsening on a background of chronicity. Chronic episodic shortness of breath is more likely to occur in asthma, hypersensitivity pneumonitis, pulmonary embolism, or cardiovascular causes.

Respiratory

- COPD.
- Asthma.
- Interstitial lung disease including IPF and sarcoidosis.
- Pleural effusion.
- Bronchiectasis/cystic fibrosis.
- Lung malignancy.
- Bronchiolitis obliterans.

Cardiovascular

- Congestive cardiac failure.
- Cardiomyopathy.
- Valvular disease.
- Pulmonary hypertension (primary and secondary).
- Shunt (intracardiac or intrapulmonary).

Other

- Neuromuscular disease.
- Anaemia.
- Thyrotoxicosis.

Assessing the patient

History, examination, and investigation will narrow down the differential diagnosis.

History

- Ask the patient to describe the character of their shortness of breath. Often they are unable to do this, but certain associated factors such as a description of chest tightness may point to the underlying problem.
- Duration and speed of onset: pneumothorax and pulmonary embolus are the usual causes of instantaneous shortness of breath.

- Usual exercise tolerance. It is helpful to ask the patient about their normal functional status. Are they breathless at the top of one flight of stairs? Also, how does this compare with 1 week or 6 months ago? This will give information on whether there is likely to be an underlying lung disease and the speed of onset of their condition.
- Severity of dyspnoea.
- Explore associated features such as wheeze, peripheral oedema, fever, cough, haemoptysis, or chest pain. If pleuritic pain consider pneumothorax, PE, or pneumonia, compared with retrosternal chest pain which may make pulmonary oedema a more likely diagnosis. In acute dyspnoea associated with wheeze, the presence of urticaria may help differentiate between anaphylaxis and asthma.
- Exacerbating features or triggers, such as cold or exercise with asthma, orthopnoea, and nocturnal breathlessness with left ventricular failure. Breathlessness on swimming or in the bath is commonly associated with diaphragmatic paralysis.
- Past medical and family history of chest disease.
- Review smoking history, drug use, occupational history, and other exposure history.
- Review medications. Has the patient stopped or run out of usual medication or been started on new medication such as beta-blockers or NSAIDs that may aggravate underlying asthma?
- In older patients with more complex medical histories the onset of dyspnoea may well be multifactorial and not simply due to a single disease process.

Examination

- Note respiratory rate, pattern of breathing, use of accessory muscles, and paradoxical abdominal movement (in diaphragmatic paralysis).
- Examine for clubbing, cyanosis, asterixis, lymphadenopathy, and evidence of SVCO (facial swelling, distended neck veins, collaterals over chest wall). Examine legs for swelling and or tenderness.
- Full examination of cardiovascular and respiratory systems.

Investigations

- SaO_2.
- Peak flow.
- FBC.
- CXR.
- ABG.
- ECG.

Consider further investigations as appropriate:

- Further blood tests (such as TFTs, cardiac enzymes, vasculitic screen, etc.).
- Exercise oximetry (e.g. 6 minute walk test).
- CT chest (HRCT/CTPA).
- Plasma BNP in the investigation of cardiac failure.
- Pulmonary function tests (± reversibility testing).
- Echocardiogram.
- Coronary angiography.

Chapter 3

Wheeze and dyspnoea

Introduction

A wheeze is a continuous musical sound that may be mono- or polyphonic in nature, depending on its cause, and may originate from an airway of any size. It is produced by oscillation of opposing walls of a narrowed airway and is typically described in expiration. Stridor is the term used for an inspiratory noise, most commonly over the central airways, and is discussed in ➲ Chapter 40.

The most common causes of acute wheeze and dyspnoea are airway diseases such as asthma and COPD; however, there is a large differential diagnosis to be considered. A useful approach is to divide the causes of wheeze and dyspnoea as to whether they occur in the upper or lower airway.

Causes of wheeze and dyspnoea

Upper airway

- Anaphylaxis: abrupt onset of wheeze and dyspnoea with urticaria and/or angioedema. Often history of insect bite or consumption of food or drug. May have had prior episodes or a positive family history.
- Epiglottitis: more commonly causes stridor and drooling. Sore throat out of proportion to visible pharyngitis. ❶ Urgent referral to ENT.
- Inducible laryngeal obstruction (ILO): Severe symptoms in absence of increased A–a gradient. Lack of response to bronchodilators. Variable flow–volume loops. Paradoxical movement of vocal cords on laryngoscopy during wheezing. ❶ Can co-exist with asthma.
- Malignancy: more commonly associated with stridor.

Lower airway

- Asthma: episodic, triggering factors, family history, history of atopy/allergy. Responds to bronchodilators.
- COPD: SOB on exertion, may have chronic productive cough, smoking history, irreversible airflow obstruction on spirometry.
- Pulmonary oedema: History of cardiac disease, chest pain, cardiac risk factors. Orthopnoea and PND.
- Bronchiectasis: Chronic productive purulent cough, episodes of fever or recurrent infections. Coarse crackles present in addition to wheeze. Crackles often inspiratory and expiratory and do not change on coughing.
- Allergic bronchopulmonary aspergillosis: deterioration in asthmatic patient. Associated eosinophilia (typically >0.5×10^9/L) with raised total and IgE against *A. fumigatus*. Segmental or lobar collapse may be seen on CXR.
- Cystic fibrosis: likely to be a known diagnosis but can present later in adulthood. Clubbed, bronchiectasis, progressive obstructive lung disease. May have associated pancreatic insufficiency with low BMI and failure to thrive. There may be family history.
- Malignancy: particularly with unilateral wheeze. May be associated with haemoptysis, smoking history, and CXR changes (particularly lobar collapse if airway obstruction is present).
- Lymphangitis carcinomatosis—Either in patient with known malignancy or occasionally as first presentation of malignancy. Abnormal CXR.
- Carcinoid syndrome—episodic flushing and diarrhoea associated with wheeze. Check 24-hour urinary 5-HIAA.
- Parasitic infection—history of travel to endemic area. Associated fever, weight loss, and peripheral blood eosinophilia. Stool and blood serology for diagnosis.

History and examination

- Episodic wheezing, often associated with dyspnoea and cough, should direct the diagnosis towards asthma. Symptoms should respond to inhaled or nebulised bronchodilators.
- Review exacerbating or triggering factors.
- Acute onset of nocturnal dyspnoea associated with wheeze may represent pulmonary oedema. Associated chest pain or cardiac risk factors may provide additional clues, as may evidence of peripheral oedema.
- Unilateral monophonic wheeze should raise suspicion of airway obstruction, for example by foreign body or malignancy.
- Past medical (including past chest) history and family history (especially for asthma).
- Smoking and drug history, occupational or recreational exposure history, and medications.
- Visual examination of upper airway should be performed along with palpation of neck for extra-thoracic obstruction and examination of the cardiac and respiratory systems.

Investigations

Initial

- SaO_2.
- HR, RR, temperature, blood pressure.
- Peak flow.
- FBC.
- CXR.
- ECG.
- ABG if SaO_2 <92%, or in COPD and concerns about hypercapnia.
- Simple spirometry if available.

Later investigation as applicable

- Pulmonary function tests.
- Plasma BNP or ECHO.
- CT chest.

Initial management

- Oxygen to maintain appropriate target oxygen saturations.
- Nebulised bronchodilator.
- Consider oral steroid.
- Consider adrenaline (IM) if evidence of anaphylaxis.
- Treatment of underlying cause.

Chapter 4

Dyspnoea in specific situations

Dyspnoea in the post-operative patient

May be due to:

- Exacerbation of an existing condition, such as asthma or COPD.
- A new condition, e.g. cardiac arrhythmia.
- The operation itself, particularly with upper GI or thoracic surgery.
- Anaesthesia and immobility.

The initial assessment of the patient should be aimed at resuscitation and treatment, particularly the need for ITU care and ventilation.

Causes

Immediate

Exclude upper airway obstruction first (➔ Chapter 40).

- Pulmonary oedema: secondary to fluid overload in patients with limited myocardial reserve, ischaemic myocardial damage, arrhythmias.
- Aspiration pneumonitis: more common in intestinal obstruction and pregnancy.
- Pulmonary embolism (consider fat and air embolism).
- Anaesthetic effect or opiate excess, causing respiratory depression.

Later

- Atelectasis: particularly following abdominal and thoracic surgery. Usually within 48 hours and more common in the elderly, COPD, smokers, and obese patients. May get lobar collapse.
- Pulmonary oedema due to fluid overload or ischaemic heart disease/ arrhythmia (usually AF).
- Post-operative pneumonia: more common if aspiration/ atelectasis/ copious secretions. Often Gram-negative bacteria.
- Pulmonary embolism, particularly pelvic procedures/known malignancy/ previous VTE.
- Exacerbation of underlying pulmonary condition such as COPD.
- Anaemia.
- ARDS.
- Metabolic acidosis, usually due to acute renal failure or sepsis.

Investigations

- Routine bloods including FBC, U&E, LFT, and CRP (though CRP often elevated secondary to operation). D-dimer will not help as it will be raised post-operatively with or without thromboembolism.
- ECG.
- CXR.
- ABG.

Management

Entirely dependent on the cause.

Basal atelectasis

Appropriate analgesia to aid coughing, chest physiotherapy ± saline nebulisers to help expectoration.

Pneumonia

Treat with high-flow oxygen, fluid resuscitation if required, broad-spectrum antibiotics, and chest physiotherapy. Use antibiotics for hospital-acquired infection to cover Gram-negative organisms (➲ Chapter 23) and consider covering for aspiration.

Pulmonary embolism

If patient is hypoxic with raised alveolar–arterial (A–a) gradient (➲ Chapter 50) and no evident cause on CXR, then proceed to CTPA. Treat with full-dose LMWH if no contra-indications (will depend on surgical procedure and discussion with surgical team).

Pulmonary oedema

Treat with oxygen, diuretics ± nitrite infusion. Central line and inotropes may be required. Investigate cause: fluid overload, myocardial damage, arrhythmia. Perform ECG, consider cardiac enzymes, tight fluid balance, echocardiogram.

Respiratory failure

If there is evidence of type 2 respiratory failure with no overt cause, consider anaesthetic agents or opiate excess (trial naloxone 400 mcg IV). Calculating the A–a gradient may be helpful in distinguishing neuromuscular causes ('pump failure') from pulmonary disease impairing gas exchange (➲ Chapter 50).

Consider precipitation of myaesthenic crisis following anaesthetic agents: intubate and ventilate, send acetylcholine receptor antibodies and treat with IV immunoglobulin and plasma exchange.

Look for evidence of pre-existing pulmonary pathology such as COPD and treat appropriately.

Anaemia

Exclude any ongoing bleeding. Cross-match and transfuse.

Dyspnoea in pregnancy

Dyspnoea during pregnancy is common, with approximately 60% of women complaining of exertional dyspnoea whilst 20% report dyspnoea at rest. Both physiological and hormonal factors contribute to dyspnoea. Distinguishing this 'physiological dyspnoea' from specific coexisting conditions or disorders complicating pregnancy is essential.

Normal physiological changes in pregnancy

Anatomical changes

In normal pregnancy there is a reduction in the functional residual capacity and residual volume due to an upward movement of the diaphragm by approximately 4 cm. There is an associated increase in vital capacity; however, total lung capacity and FEV_1 remain unchanged.

Ventilation

Minute ventilation increases because of stimulation by elevated progesterone levels and the PaO_2 increases. Pregnant women usually mildly hyperventilate to maintain a low $PaCO_2$ in order to maintain a gradient for CO_2 diffusion from fetal blood. In addition, cardiac output increases by up to 40% and plasma volume by up to 50%.

Haemodynamic changes

Progressive increase in cardiac output from the first trimester; up to 40% above baseline by the third trimester.

Thrombotic state

Increased coagulation factors and venous stasis of the pelvic veins leads to a fivefold increased risk of thromboembolism, which is a major cause of maternal death.

Causes of shortness of breath in pregnancy

Pulmonary

- Exacerbation or worsening of pre-existing condition, e.g. asthma, bronchiectasis, pulmonary hypertension.
- Pulmonary embolism.
- Aspiration pneumonitis.
- Pneumothorax.
- Pleural effusion: can be seen in the post-partum period and rarely in ovarian hyperstimulation syndrome (following IVF).

Cardiac

- Valvular heart disease (may previously have been undiagnosed and precipitated by increased cardiac output).
- Undiagnosed mitral stenosis can cause pulmonary oedema in labour.
- Cardiomyopathy.

Other

- ARDS: associated with obstetric complications, e.g. amniotic fluid embolus, placental abruption, eclampsia, or non-obstetric conditions which are more common in pregnancy, e.g. gastric aspiration, sepsis (pelvic and non-pelvic), and massive haemorrhage.
- Anaemia.

Pregnancy-specific disorders

- Amniotic fluid embolization (rare, 1 in 25 000). High mortality.
- Tocolytic pulmonary oedema (caused by beta-adrenergic agonists used to inhibit pre-term labour).
- Pre-eclampsia and pulmonary oedema.
- Peri-partum cardiomyopathy (usually develops in the last month of pregnancy).

Asthma in pregnancy

Approximately a third become worse, a third become better, and a third stay the same. Asthma deterioration is often between weeks 24 and 36.

Asthma is associated with an increased risk of pre-eclampsia. However, studies have shown that increased asthma symptoms and poor control both before and during pregnancy lead to this increased risk, as opposed to asthma alone.

Asthma is also associated with an increased risk of intra-uterine growth retardation (IUGR). Again, studies have shown that those with well-controlled asthma (relatively asymptomatic, GINA 1) have no or minimal IUGR, with increasing IUGR as control or symptoms worsen.

There are often compliance issues with asthma medications during pregnancy as women are concerned about the possible effects on the fetus. Asthma medications, including oral steroids, are generally regarded as safe in pregnancy and should be continued. There is a paucity of evidence for the use of asthma biologics in pregnancy currently, however they may be continued or initiated if the risk of not doing so is deemed to outweigh the potential risks of using them.

► Poor control is more harmful to the mother and fetus than asthma medication.

Acute asthma in pregnancy

- Treat as for the non-pregnant asthmatic (➔ Chapter 20).
- GORD often a trigger factor for asthma and this increases in pregnancy.
- Maintain SaO_2 94–98% to prevent fetal hypoxia.
- Monitor fetus in severe asthma and liaise with obstetricians.

Drugs

All common asthma medications can be continued in pregnancy (beta-2 agonists, inhaled corticosteroids, long-acting beta-agonists, leukotriene receptor antagonists, theophylline) except for the newer biologic agents where there is little data to date on their use in pregnancy. However, if the mother has good control, then stopping requires careful consideration as worsening control will do more harm.

Labour

Because of increased release of endogenous steroid it is very rare to have an acute exacerbation of asthma during labour.

Prostaglandin E_2 may be safely used in induction of labour, whilst prostaglandin F_2 alpha, used in post-partum haemorrhage, may cause bronchospasm.

Use IV hydrocortisone 100 mg 6–8 hourly during labour in those who have been taking >7.5 mg oral prednisolone for >2 weeks before delivery.

Pulmonary embolism in pregnancy

Despite increased awareness, this remains the most common cause of maternal death and mortality still occurs because of lack of recognition and timely diagnosis.

There is increased risk of thromboembolism in pregnancy because of:

- increased coagulability.
- increased venous stasis: >30% reduction in flow by 15/40 weeks, >60% by 36/40 weeks.

Ileofemoral deep vein thrombosis (DVT) occurs more commonly than popliteofemoral DVT in pregnancy and is far more frequent than in the non-pregnant population. Pregnancy is also a risk factor for recurrent DVT, with a threefold increase in relative risk.

Increased risk of pulmonary embolism

- Age >35 years.
- Caesarian section.
- Increased BMI.
- Positive family history or known thrombophilia.
- Previous thrombosis.
- Pre-eclampsia.

Investigation of pulmonary embolism in pregnancy

If there is clinical suspicion of PE, D-dimer will not add to the investigation as it is usually raised in normal pregnancy (➔ Chapter 28). The negative predictive value is also less reliable in pregnancy. Ideally, the first investigation of choice should be bilateral leg USS. This involves no radiation exposure to the mother or fetus and if positive precludes the need for further investigation. The choice of further investigation is between CTPA and ventilation-perfusion scan. Radiation doses are as follows.

- Perfusion scan exposes the fetus to 0.5 mGy.
- Ventilation scan <0.35 mGy.
- CXR <0.1 mGy.

A CTPA gives a radiation dose to the fetus that is less than that of a V/Q scan, but an increased exposure to the mother which increases the lifetime risk of breast cancer in the mother by 13.6%. On the basis of this, the investigation of choice in those with a normal CXR is a perfusion scan.

Treatment of pulmonary embolism

- Requires a minimum of 3 months anticoagulation.
- Avoid warfarin: teratogenic to the fetus and increased risk of maternal haemorrhage. DOACs are also not recommended.
- Low molecular weight heparin (LMWH) with dosing based on their booking weight is the anticoagulant of choice, with a switch to unfractionated heparin for the delivery. Levels of LMWH can be monitored with anti-Xa levels (0.4–1.2 U/mL therapeutic anticoagulation).
- Anticoagulation should be continued throughout the pregnancy and for at least 6 weeks post-partum or until 3 months treatment has been completed.
- Pregnancy is not a contra-indication to thrombolysis for massive PE.

Other pre-existing pulmonary conditions in pregnancy

Pulmonary hypertension

Pregnancy occurring in those with pulmonary hypertension has an associated high mortality, up to 30–50%. Increased cardiac output precipitates right heart failure. IUGR occurs in >30%. Echocardiography does not reliably measure pulmonary artery pressure in pregnancy.

Cystic fibrosis

In those with FEV_1 >60% predicted, there is no increased mortality associated with pregnancy. In those with more severe disease the outcome is poor, with increased perinatal mortality due to pre-term delivery or complications of CF. There is a paucity of evidence for the use of CFTR modulators in pregnancy.

Lymphangioleiomyomatosis

Often presents for the first time in pregnancy; otherwise worsens in pregnancy as the disease process (abnormal proliferation of smooth muscle cells) is driven by oestrogen. Common presentations include dyspnoea, cough, pneumothorax, and pleural effusion (particularly chylothorax).

Dyspnoea and fever in the returning traveller

Both travel abroad by UK residents and the number of visitors and immigrants from abroad are increasing year by year, and therefore this is becoming an increasingly common presentation to A&E. Approximately half of those presenting after recent travel will have a non-tropical cause for their fever and shortness of breath (e.g. community-acquired pneumonia). In returning travellers from tropical areas, malaria is by far the most common cause of fever. Cause of infection is dependent on the location and duration of travel. Differential diagnosis can be further narrowed down by considering exposure history, relevant incubation period, and findings.

History

- Country travelled to and stopovers.
- Duration of travel.
- Accommodation, i.e. hotel, camping.
- Food and water consumed, i.e. fresh, bottled, tinned.
- Any insect or animal bites.
- Domestic pets.
- Leisure activities, e.g. watersports.
- Occupation.
- Vaccinations and prophylaxis.
- Sexual activity, IV drug use, tattooing, transfusions.
- Contacts with unwell people.
- PMH.

Examination

Full systemic examination.

Look in particular for skin and genital lesions, conjunctival change, lymphadenopathy, liver, and spleen.

Investigations

- FBC, U&E, LFTs, CRP.
- Thick and thin films, blood antigen detection testing for malaria.
- Serology.
- Urinalysis and MSU.
- Blood cultures.
- Stool culture if appropriate.
- CXR.
- Further imaging: USS/CT.
- Specific tests for a suspected diagnosis: antibody titres, immunological investigations.

Causes

More frequent

- Community-acquired pneumonia.
- Mycoplasma.
    - Atypical pneumonia. Often presents with dry cough, headache, diarrhoea, anaemia (cold agglutinin), and abnormal LFT.

- *Legionella.*
  - Outbreaks in hotels with contaminated cooling systems.
  - Incubation 2–10 days.
  - Prodromal viral-like illness; then dry cough, tachypnoea, diarrhoea, and confusion.
  - Lymphopaenia and hyponatraemia seen.
  - Diagnosis: urinary *Legionella* antigen ± serology.
  - Treatment with macrolides ± rifampicin.
- Tuberculosis.
  - Contact history, often productive cough with fevers, sweats, and weight loss. Abnormal CXR. Be aware of extrapulmonary tuberculosis.
- Typhoid.
  - Insidious onset with headache and fever, then cough, rash (rose-spots), and constipation. Later get diarrhoea, pneumonia, and other complications.
  - Diagnosis: blood cultures early, urine and stool cultures later.
  - Treatment with ciprofloxacin.
- Viral pneumonia including COVID-19.

Less common

- Q fever.
  - Caused by *Coxiella burnetii.* Infection by inhalation (increased risk with farmyard exposure). Incubation 2–3 weeks.
  - Fever, myalgia, dry cough, GI symptoms, and chest pain. 30–50% develop pneumonia.
  - Diagnosis on serology. Treat with doxycycline.
- Diphtheria.
  - Epidemic in Russia and Eastern Europe.
  - Incubation 2–5 days.
  - Laryngeal diphtheria gives husky voice, cough, and later dyspnoea and stridor due to respiratory obstruction. Usually cervical lymph nodes (giving 'bull neck') and pharyngeal membrane (greyish yellow) present.
  - Diagnosis usually clinical (send cultures and serology). Treat with anti-toxin and macrolide or penicillin.
- Pertussis.
  - 90% of cases occur in children <5 years of age but can affect any age.
  - Initially malaise, then characteristic paroxysms of coughing; 'whoop' characteristically in children.
  - Diagnosis by culture of nasopharyngeal secretions, PCR, or serology; treat with macrolides.
- Anthrax.
  - Occurs worldwide.
  - Transmission through direct contact with infected animals.
  - Inhalation of spores results in dry cough and fever with chest discomfort for 2–3 days; then dramatic deterioration with dyspnoea and hypoxia.
  - CXR shows widened mediastinum (due to haemorrhagic mediastinitis) or pleural effusion.
  - Diagnosed by culture (Gram-positive rod), PCR, or fourfold antibody rise. Treat with penicillin or macrolides, drain pleural fluid.

- Tularaemia.
    - Worldwide, but frequently seen in the USA.
    - Transmission via handling infected meat or tick bite.
    - Pneumonic form.
    - Diagnose on culture or serology and treat with gentamicin.
- Melioidosis.
    - Penetrates skin abrasions: usually seen in those who go barefoot, e.g. paddy-field farmers in Southeast Asia.
    - Acute septicaemia with lung, kidney, and liver involvement or chronic pneumonic form. CXR may resemble TB.
    - Diagnose on culture; treat with ceftazidime.
- Botulism.
    - *Clostridium botulinum* proliferates in preserved canned foods.
    - Toxins cause neuromuscular blockade, with neurological symptoms dominating and respiratory insufficiency occurring.
    - Toxin detected in serum or faeces.
    - Anti-toxin and supportive treatment.
- Brucellosis.
    - Worldwide zoonosis.
    - Infection through unpasteurised milk.
    - Usually undulating fever, malaise, and night sweats. Localised brucellosis in the lung (with systemic symptoms in a third) is uncommon.
    - Diagnose on culture or serology. Treat with doxycycline and rifampicin.

Chapter 5

Cough, sputum, and fever

Cough, sputum, and fever

The development of the combination of a cough, sputum production, and a fever usually implies pulmonary infection of some form. It may be a new infection in otherwise normal lungs, e.g. pneumonia, or the worsening of a chronic disease, e.g. bronchiectasis or COPD. The assessment of the patient follows the standard format.

History

A full history should be taken from the patient and/or relatives as soon as the situation is sufficiently stable to do so.

- Cough: acute/chronic.
- Sputum.
  - Acute/chronic, able to expectorate, purulent, associated haemoptysis.
  - If chronic, what is normal volume, colour, consistency?
  - Streaky haemoptysis common in CF and bronchiectasis.
- Other symptoms.
  - Dyspnoea, chest pain, wheeze, malaise, weight loss.
- Previous medical history.
  - Prior cardiorespiratory disease.
  - Immunosuppression: disease-related or iatrogenic.
- Prior medications.
  - May indicate chronic respiratory disease.
  - Prior antibiotic use: determine which antibiotics have previously improved symptoms. If previous lack of response to oral antibiotics, consider *Pseudomonas* infection.
- Allergies.
  - Penicillin allergy and if present its nature. Many patients with 'penicillin allergy' will be able to tolerate cephalosporins.
- Travel.
  - Risks for TB, *Legionella*.
- Vaccination history.
- Smoking.
- Alcohol.
- Pets: in particular whether the patient keeps birds.
- Family history.

Examination

- General.
  - How unwell is the patient? The initial end of the bed assessment of the acute patient should guide subsequent actions.
- Respiratory.
  - Airway.
  - Respiratory rate and effort.
  - Cyanosis: peripheral or central.
  - Evidence of chronic lung disease, e.g. hyperinflation, clubbing.
  - Expansion, percussion, auscultation. Presence of secretions, consolidation or pleural fluid.
- Circulation.
  - Evidence of sepsis (hypotension, tachycardia).

- Urine output and fluid balance.
- Neurological assessment.
  - Look for reasons for aspiration pneumonia: depressed conscious level, dysphasia, dysphagia, stroke, neuromuscular disease. If suspected, the patient should remain nil by mouth until formal assessment is possible.

Investigations

- Temperature, heart rate, blood pressure, respiratory rate.
- Oxygen saturation.
- Blood glucose.
- ECG.
- Bloods including FBC (note WCC including eosinophils), U&Es, LFTs.
- CRP.
- Clotting screen: coagulopathy of sepsis or DIC.
- Blood cultures prior to antibiotics.
- CXR.
- Arterial blood gas.
- Sputum cultures in:
  - Chronic respiratory disease where bacterial pathogen is uncertain or when antibiotic resistance is suspected, e.g. CF and bronchiectasis.
  - Suspected TB (three samples for AFB).
- Viral nose/throat swab for PCR.
- Urinary antigen tests to identify bacterial antigens in urine. They can provide rapid results, helping guide diagnosis and therapy even if performed after the initiation of antibiotic therapy. There are two commonly performed tests.

Legionella urinary antigen

- Most *Legionella* pneumonia (80%) is caused by *Legionella pneumophila* serogroup 1. *Legionella* pneumonia is more likely to cause severe community-acquired pneumonia (CAP).
- Some laboratories only test for serogroup 1 and so it is important to know what test your local laboratory uses as a negative result does not exclude *Legionella*.

Pneumococcal urinary antigen

- *Streptococcus pneumoniae* antigen can be detected in the urine.
  - Individual hospitals will have their own policies for use of these tests. The BTS recommends both *Legionella* urinary antigen and pneumococcal urinary antigen are performed in severe community-acquired pneumonia.
- Serology for atypical pathogens.
  - Change in IgG and IgM titre in paired blood samples (taken when ill and convalescing) can prove infection.
  - *Legionella pneumophila*, *Mycoplasma*, and *Chlamydia pneumoniae* are the usual pathogens tested for.
  - No use in initial management of the acutely unwell patient in whom urinary antigen testing is preferred.
  - Criteria for performing these tests depend on the requirement for microbiological surveillance and are usually agreed locally between clinicians, laboratory staff, and public health officers.

- Diagnostic pleural aspiration if a pleural effusion is present.
  - Check fluid pH, protein, LDH, glucose, MC & S, AFBs.
- Bronchoscopy.
  - Rarely needed in the acute setting for diagnosis. It should be considered in the immunocompromised (if they are stable enough for it to be done safely), as the potential pathogens are more varied, or if aspiration of a foreign body is suspected.

Differential diagnosis

- Pneumonia.
  - Bacterial.
  - Viral including COVID-19.
  - Fungal.
- Acute bronchitis.
- Acute exacerbation of COPD.
- Acute exacerbation of known bronchiectasis/CF.
- Mycobacterial disease.
  - TB.
  - Non-tuberculous *Mycobacterium*.
- Cryptogenic organising pneumonia (COP).
- Eosinophilic pneumonia.
- Hypersensitivity pneumonitis.
- Allergic bronchopulmonary aspergillosis (ABPA).

Management

Severity assessment

Initial care should be guided by:
- Heart rate, blood pressure, respiratory rate, temperature.
- Oxygen saturation.
- ABG: oxygenation, ventilation, and tissue perfusion via serum lactate.
- Neurological status: GCS, confusion.
- Circulation and intravascular volume status.

In community-acquired pneumonia there are several proposed severity assessment scores. The CURB-65 score is described in ➔ Chapter 23.

The basis of the treatment of pneumonia and other forms of pulmonary infection follows the basic scheme for all acute scenarios. It consists of:

- The immediate recognition of any life-threatening conditions and their prompt correction (➔ Chapter 1).
- ABC approach.
- Oxygen: ensure adequate arterial levels to help maintain O_2 delivery to the tissues.
  - Most patients with pneumonia have type 1 respiratory failure, but may present with acute type 2 respiratory failure (➔ Chapter 8). They are best helped by providing a FiO_2 that maintains an adequate arterial oxygen level. Acute hypercapnia and respiratory acidosis with a normal base excess implies acute ventilatory failure and should prompt consideration of ICU care.

    - Limiting the FiO_2 may be appropriate for some COPD patients for whom oxygen genuinely does depress minute ventilation. An acute respiratory acidosis should be closely monitored alongside maximal therapy and assisted ventilation considered.
- Consider NIV (➲ Chapter 44).
- Treat underlying condition:
    - Pneumonia–follow BTS guidelines (➲ Chapter 23).
    - Exacerbation of COPD (➲ Chapter 21).
    - Exacerbation of bronchiectasis (➲ Chapter 30).
    - Exacerbation of CF (➲ Chapter 31).
    - Immunocompromised (➲ Chapter 13).
- Regular observations.
    - Assess response to therapy with monitoring of temperature, blood pressure, heart rate, oxygen saturation, and urine output. Can be used as 'early warning scores'.
- Nutrition.
- Physiotherapy.
    - Effective airway clearance is crucial in bronchiectasis (➲ Chapter 30).

Chapter 6

Haemoptysis

Haemoptysis

Haemoptysis refers to the expectoration of blood or blood-stained sputum.

Causes

Respiratory

- Bronchial carcinoma.
- Pneumonia.
- Tuberculosis.
- Cystic fibrosis.
- Bronchiectasis.
- Aspergilloma.

Vascular/CVS

- Pulmonary embolism.
- Mitral stenosis.
- Arteriovenous malformation.
- Hereditary haemorrhagic telangiectasia.
- Pulmonary oedema.

Iatrogenic

- Post-bronchoscopy.
- Post-instrumentation.

Vasculitis

- Granulomatosis with polyangiitis (GPA).
- Anti-glomerular basement membrane (anti-GBM) disease—Goodpasture's syndrome.

Other

- Invading oesophageal carcinoma or metastatic disease.
- Clotting disorders.
- Anti-coagulant or antiplatelet medication.
- Endometriosis.
- Upper airway origin of blood (epistaxis, bleeding gums, upper airway malignancy).

History

- Is it blood alone or blood mixed with sputum? Colour of sputum?
    - Pulmonary oedema classically pink frothy sputum. Bronchiectasis and pneumonia usually present with blood mixed with sputum.
- Chronicity of symptoms/previous episodes.
    - Points towards chronic condition, e.g. bronchiectasis, CF.
- Amount of blood.
    - Aspergilloma, vasculitis, AVM, CF, invading cancer most likely to cause massive haemoptysis.
- Time of occurrence of haemoptysis.
    - Occurring particularly after lying down is suggestive of an upper airway origin. Occurring with menstruation is suggestive of endometriosis.
- Associated symptoms.
    - Acute SOB and chest pain makes pneumonia or pulmonary embolism more likely, although SOB alone points toward pulmonary oedema. Progressive SOB more suggestive of mitral stenosis.

  - Fevers associated with weight loss occur in TB, although weight loss without fever may indicate lung cancer.
- Other sites of bleeding.
  - Haematuria occurring in vasculitis.
  - Epistaxis suggestive of GPA or hereditary haemorrhagic telangiectasia.
- Thorough PMH, travel, and drug history.

Examination

Inspection

- Cachexia: TB, cancer.
- Clubbing: bronchiectasis, lung cancer.
- Nasal passages (crusting) and saddling of nose in GPA.
- Malar flush.
- Telangiectasia.
- Raised JVP, peripheral oedema.
- Swollen face and distended veins in SVCO associated with cancer.
- Scars: previous surgery for lung cancer or bronchiectasis, chest drain scars.

Palpation

- Pulse rate and rhythm: tachycardia associated with infection and PE; AF and anti-coagulation associated with mitral stenosis.
- Lymphadenopathy: infection (particularly TB) and cancer.
- Calf swelling and tenderness.

Auscultation

- Crackles: generally fine inspiratory with pulmonary oedema; coarse with infection or bronchiectasis.
- Bronchial breathing: infection.
- Decreased breath sounds/dull percussion note: effusion may point to cancer, TB, or pneumonia, cardiac failure (more commonly bilateral), or pulmonary embolism.
- Diastolic murmur of mitral stenosis.

Investigations

- FBC.
- U&E.
- Clotting screen.
- Urine dip (proteinuria and haematuria in vasculitis).
- ECG.
- CXR.
- Arterial blood gas if SaO_2 <95%.
- Sputum for MC&S (and AFBs if suspected).
- ESR/CRP.

Specific investigations

- ANCA and antiglomerular basement membrane antibody if vasculitis suspected.
- *Aspergillus* precipitins (strongly positive in aspergilloma) and specific IgE to *Aspergillus*.
- Bronchoscopy.

- CT chest: type dependent on suspicion (discuss with radiologist) to investigate PE, cancer, AVM, bronchiectasis.
- Echocardiography if investigating mitral stenosis or pulmonary hypertension as the suspected cause of haemoptysis.

Management

- ABC.
- IV access (large bore if massive haemoptysis).
- Bloods including FBC, renal function, liver function, and clotting. Urgent cross-match if massive haemoptysis.
- Reverse anticoagulants.
- CXR.
- CT angiogram of the chest if large-volume haemoptysis.

Small-volume haemoptysis

- As above.
- Start antibiotics if evidence of infection (low threshold in those with bronchiectasis and CF).
- Consider oral tranexamic acid (15–25 mg/kg tds, max. 1 g tds).
- CT chest ± bronchoscopy and further investigations as appropriate.

Massive haemoptysis (100–600 ml in 24 hours)

- Manage as above.
- High-flow oxygen.
- IV crystalloids.
- If known which lung the blood is coming from (such as post-bronchoscopy or instrumentation) then nurse patient with bleeding lung down.
- Adrenaline nebuliser (5 ml of 1:1000).
- Bronchoscopy is rarely useful in the acute massive bleed. Fibreoptic bronchoscopy has no role; occasionally rigid bronchoscopy (usually performed by thoracic surgeons) will allow clot removal or haemostasis.
- Selective bronchial angiography and embolisation. Tertiary service. Source of bleeding difficult to determine but dilated tortuous vessels embolised (>2.5 mm). Spinal artery thrombosis potential complication.
- IV terlipressin (2 mg STAT then 1–2 mg every 4–6 hours) or less commonly vasopressin can sometimes be used until bleeding settles.
- Urgent referral to ITU may be required. They may consider intubating with a double lumen ET tube.
- Surgical resection may be considered as a last resort.

In palliative cases with massive haemoptysis the above management may not be appropriate. Use high-flow oxygen and consider midazolam to alleviate distressing symptoms.

Chapter 7

Chest pain

Chest pain

There are many causes of chest pain, both respiratory and non-respiratory. Differentiating between them relies on a thorough history and examination, giving rise to diagnosis by pattern recognition, as well as appropriate investigations.

Causes

Respiratory

Lung parenchyma

- Pneumonia: associated with fever, rigors, sputum production. Consolidation on CXR.
- Malignancy: either associated with a complication such as infection, effusion, or PE, or due to invasion of chest wall.
- Sarcoid: cough and SOB. Review skin, joint, or eye problems.

Pleura

- Pneumothorax: sudden-onset pleuritic pain and SOB. Young tall male smokers are at increased risk of primary spontaneous pneumothorax.
- Pleural effusion.
- Pleurisy: consider viral, drug-induced, SLE, familial Mediterranean fever.

Pulmonary vasculature

- Pulmonary embolus: pleuritic pain, SOB, haemoptysis, and risk factors (particularly pregnancy). PIOPED study found 97% presented with pain, SOB, or tachycardia, with 90% presenting with SOB, tachycardia, or DVT.

Cardiac

- Ischaemic heart disease: classic story. Worse on exertion/relieved with rest, radiates to jaw/arm. Associated with sweating, nausea, SOB. Cardiac risk factors. Consider coronary artery vasospasm in those with a history of recent cocaine use with cardiac-sounding chest pain.
- Aortic dissection: sudden severe ripping pain. More common in older men. Risk factors include hypertension and less commonly Marfan's syndrome, aortic coarctation, and rarely pregnancy. Check pulses, asymmetrical BP readings in arms, murmur of aortic regurgitation, ischaemic ECG, widened mediastinum on CXR.
- Pericarditis: pain reduced on sitting forward. Listen for rub. ECG: widespread 'saddle-shaped' ST elevation.
- Valvular heart disease: particularly aortic stenosis. Progressive angina, dyspnoea, and syncope.

Gastro-intestinal

- Gastro-oesophageal reflux: burning pain, radiates to back and jaw. Worse after meals or on lying. Is it relieved by antacids?.
- Mediastinitis: Boerhaeve's syndrome (oesophageal rupture after vomiting), iatrogenic, caustic substance ingestion, and Barrett's oesophagus. Air in mediastinum on CXR. Usually unwell.
- Pancreatitis, biliary colic.
- PUD.

Chest wall

- Musculoskeletal: insidious, long history, associated trauma or recent repetitive activity. Worse on movement and inspiration.
- Fractured rib.
- Costochondritis (Tietze's syndrome).
- Autoimmune disease (SLE, rheumatoid involving thoracic joints).
- Skin and sensory nerves, e.g. shingles.

History

Pain

- Nature: respiratory pain is typically pleuritic, whilst most cardiac causes of pain have characteristic patterns.
- Site.
- Severity.
- Duration.
- Radiation.
- Exacerbating or relieving factors (e.g. pain associated with pericarditis eases with leaning forward).
- Similar pain in past.

Other features

- Associated symptoms: cough, fever, sputum production, haemoptysis, SOB, nausea, sweating.
- Risk factors: recent travel, immobility, trauma, cardiac risk factors.
- Past medical history and family history.

Examination

- Observations: temperature, oxygen saturations, heart rate, blood pressure, respiratory rate.
- Chest wall tenderness does not exclude an underlying cause of chest pain.
- Examine for associated features of disease:
  - Rashes, ulcers, arthritis in autoimmune conditions.
  - Clubbing, cachexia, and lymphadenopathy in lung cancer.
- Auscultation and percussion of chest.
- Listen for pericardial rubs.
- Examine abdomen.

Investigations

- FBC.
- U&Es (severity scoring in pneumonia).
- LFTs and amylase if concerns about GI pathology.
- Inflammatory markers.
- D-dimer: if low or intermediate suspicion of PE (high negative predictive value).
- High sensitivity troponin—ESC recommends at 0h and 1h post-onset of pain.
- ECG.
- CXR.
- ABG (if oxygen saturations <92%).

Further investigations as appropriate

- CTPA (or V/Q) if D-dimer positive, no alternative diagnosis more likely, or high clinical suspicion of PE (➲ Chapter 28).
- ECHO for investigation of cardiac causes.
- Focused pleural ultrasound +/– diagnostic pleural aspiration.
- Serum autoantibodies.
- CT chest.
- Bone scan.

Chapter 8

Respiratory failure

Acute hypoxaemic respiratory failure

Type 1 respiratory failure occurs in the presence of a po_2 <8 kPa with a normal or low $Paco_2$. This is most commonly caused by a ventilation–perfusion mismatch at the alveolar level, with an increase in the alveolar–arterial (A–a) gradient (see below). It is hard to differentiate between acute and chronic hypoxaemic respiratory failure on blood gases alone; other markers such as polycythaemia and cor pulmonale point to chronicity.

Causes of acute type 1 respiratory failure

Pulmonary

- Asthma.
- Pneumonia.
- Pneumothorax.
- Exacerbation of pre-existing pulmonary disease (COPD, bronchiectasis, interstitial lung disease).
- Pulmonary haemorrhage.

Vascular

- Pulmonary embolism.
- Cardiogenic pulmonary oedema.
- Intra-cardiac shunt.
- AV malformation in the lung.
- Pulmonary arterial hypertension.

Upper airway

- Acute epiglottitis.
- Tumour or foreign body.

Pathophysiology

Acute hypoxaemic respiratory failure occurs in the presence of a ventilation–perfusion mismatch or shunting. With a mismatch, areas of underventilated lung which are still adequately perfused cause hypoxaemia, whilst in shunting, either intrapulmonary or intracardiac, mixed venous blood bypasses ventilated lung. In both cases the A–a oxygen difference (usually <2 kPa) is increased. An increase in the A–a oxygen gradient indicates pulmonary disease to be the cause of hypoxia.

$$\text{A} - \text{a gradient} = \text{PaO}_2 - \left(\text{PaO}_2 + \text{PaCO}_2/0.8\right)$$

where A indicates alveolar (% inspired oxygen of 100 – 7, i.e. if breathing air 21% of (100 – 7) ≈ 20 kPa), a indicates arterial, and 0.8 is the respiratory quotient (➔ Chapter 50 for more detailed explanation).

Even in the normal lung, not all alveoli are optimally perfused and ventilated. In general the apices are relatively underperfused compared with the bases because of the effects of gravity on pulmonary blood flow.

Alveoli that are optimally perfused but not adequately ventilated are called low V/Q units and act like a shunt. Low V/Q units may occur because of either underventilation secondary to a pathological process in the airway or interstitium or relative overperfusion, such as in pulmonary embolism, with diversion of blood away from the parts of the lung where flow is obstructed by emboli.

A shunt is present where hypoxia cannot be corrected despite the administration of 100% inhaled oxygen. Pulmonary shunts occur in the presence of pneumonia, atelectasis, and severe pulmonary oedema, whilst vascular shunts occur in atrial and ventricular septal defects, patent ductus arteriosus or foramen ovale, or an arteriovenous malformation in the lung.

Clinical assessment

History

- Features of infection such as cough, fever, sputum production, or pleuritic chest pain. Possibility of aspiration.
- PMH of cardiac or valvular disease. History of chest pain, increasing shortness of breath on exertion, or orthopnoea and paroxysmal nocturnal dyspnoea.
- Unilateral leg swelling; history of immobility or recent surgery. Previous thromboembolism.
- Known pulmonary disease.
- Drug history (particularly possible pulmonary toxic drugs), environmental exposure.

Examination

On observation the patient is likely to be dyspnoeic and may be cyanosed. Evidence of cor pulmonale may point to chronicity. Stridor indicates an upper respiratory airway problem, whilst audible wheeze is suggestive of asthma or COPD.

Examine for valvular heart disease and percuss/auscultate chest to identify effusion, pneumothorax, or consolidation. Look for peripheral oedema, calf swelling, and signs of associated disease such as clubbing, rheumatoid joints, and skin rashes.

Investigation

- FBC to investigate for polycythaemia. U&Es, cardiac enzymes.
- CXR.
- ABG.
- ECG—acute right heart strain is suggestive of large pulmonary embolus.
- Further investigation as appropriate:
  - Pulmonary function testing.
  - CT chest/CTPA
  - ECHO.
  - Autoimmune screen.

Management

- Ensure airway is patent and safe.
  - If stridor is present seek an urgent ENT opinion.
  - Consider intubation if concerns.
- Correct hypoxaemia with high-flow oxygen. Aim to maintain oxygen saturations >92%. If hypoxaemia cannot be corrected with oxygen alone then consider CPAP if appropriate, or intubation and ventilation.
- Discuss with ITU, particularly if requiring high-percentage oxygen maintain oxygen levels.
- Treat the underlying cause.

Acute hypercapnic respiratory failure

Type 2 respiratory failure occurs when there is a low PaO_2 (<8 kPa) in the presence of a raised CO_2 level (>6 kPa). Hypercapnic respiratory failure is the end result of many causes of respiratory failure (e.g. pneumonia, pulmonary oedema), not just chronic lung conditions such as COPD. It results from an overall reduction in ventilation (alveolar hypoventilation), an increase in the proportion of dead-space ventilation, or an imbalance between load and capacity.

Causes

Reduction in minute ventilation

- Neuromuscular disorders affecting the respiratory muscles, such as muscular dystrophy, motor neuron disease, myasthenia gravis, and Guillain–Barré syndrome.
- CNS depression
  - Drug overdose.
  - Vascular abnormality or tumour affecting the brainstem.
  - Hypothyroidism.
- Chest wall abnormalities (such as severe kyphoscoliosis).
- Morbid obesity (causing obesity hypoventilation syndrome)—increasingly common.

Increased dead-space ventilation

- Obstructive airways disease, such as COPD, asthma, and CF.
- Upper airway causes such as tracheal tumours and epiglottitis.

Alveolar abnormalities

Hypercapnia may also occur in cases of hypoxaemic respiratory failure where diffuse alveolar filling initially causes shunting and increased work of breathing; however, with time this may lead to decreased alveolar ventilation. Examples of this include severe pulmonary oedema, pneumonia, and pulmonary haemorrhage.

Acute versus chronic

This can be determined from the blood gases. In acute conditions, e.g. asthma and pneumonia, hypercapnia will be associated with acidosis and a normal bicarbonate. In conditions with chronic hypercapnia, the bicarbonate will be raised because of renal compensation. Acidosis may or may not be present depending on the degree of acute respiratory compromise.

Other factors that suggest chronicity include evidence of right heart strain and cor pulmonale.

Assessment

- Full history including:
  - Prior chest problems.
  - Muscle weakness, swallowing difficulties, change in speech.
  - Breathlessness on lying flat or swimming (suggestive of diaphragmatic paralysis).
  - Drug history.
- Examine for evidence of associated pathology:
  - Chest wall abnormalities such as kyphosis or scoliosis.

- Muscle wasting or fasciculation.
- Signs of hyperinflation/prolonged expiratory phase (obstructive airways disease).
- Features of drug overdose such as pinpoint pupils with opiates.
- Paradoxical abdominal movement on breathing.

Investigations

- Routine bloods to include TFTs.
- CXR.
- ABG.
- ECG (for evidence of right heart strain).
- Lung function tests, including where necessary:
    - Lying and standing VC if concerns regarding neuromuscular involvement.
    - SNIP (inspiratory pressure) to investigate diaphragmatic weakness).

Further management

- First ensure a safe airway and check breathing and circulation.
- Establish IV access.
- Commence treatment for underlying cause, e.g. nebulised bronchodilators, diuretics.
- Ongoing management will depend on cause of hypercapnia.
    - *Acute condition*, e.g. asthma, pneumonia: discussion with ITU for consideration of ventilation (if appropriate). If pulmonary oedema—CPAP or invasive ventilation may be appropriate.
    - *Chronic condition*, e.g. COPD/neuromuscular disease/obesity hypoventilation: controlled oxygen, monitoring CO_2. May need NIV or invasive ventilation (➔ Chapter 44).

! Cor pulmonale

Cor pulmonale describes the cardiovascular consequences of chronic hypoxia resulting from chronic lung disease, usually referring to a combination of pulmonary hypertension and fluid retention. Chronic hypoxaemia, often in association with hypercapnia, results in progressive pulmonary hypertension and right ventricular remodelling (hypertrophy and dilatation). Although right ventricular output is often maintained, right ventricular failure may occur over time.

Diagnosis

- Chronic hypoxic lung disease (+ hypercapnia usually).
- Pulmonary hypertension.
- Fluid retention.

Pulmonary hypertension

Pulmonary hypertension (defined in cor pulmonale as a resting pulmonary artery pressure (PAP) >20 mmHg) is thought to arise as a result of pulmonary vascular bed remodelling in response to chronic alveolar hypoxia (distinct from acute vasoconstriction secondary to acute hypoxia). Associated hypercapnic acidosis and polycythaemia (secondary to hypoxia) may also contribute to increased pulmonary pressures.

Fluid retention

Fluid retention is not usually the result of right heart failure *per se* (as cardiac output in cor pulmonale is maintained), but rather occurs through renal retention of salt and water in a neurohormonal response to hypoxaemia. Thus peripheral oedema may arise in the absence of a truly 'failing' right ventricle, as capillary permeability increases in response to the associated hypercapnic state.

Causes

Three major groups of respiratory disease cause cor pulmonale; the majority (estimated around 80%) are due to obstructive lung disease. The following list excludes pulmonary vascular disease (primary pulmonary hypertension, chronic thrombo-emboli, veno-occlusive disease). Asterisks indicate more common causes.

Obstructive lung disease

- COPD.*
- Asthma (+ irreversible airways obstruction).
- Bronchiectasis.
- CF.
- Obliterative bronchiolitis.

Restrictive lung disease

- Kyphoscoliosis.*
- Fibrotic interstitial lung disease (e.g. idiopathic pulmonary fibrosis)
- Neuromuscular disease (myopathies, diaphragm paralysis).
- Post pulmonary TB (fibrosis, pleural thickening, thoracoplasty).
- Pneumoconiosis.

Breathing pattern dysfunction

- Obstructive sleep apnoea.*

- Obesity hypoventilation syndrome.
- Any cause of chronic 'central' hypoventilation (syringobulbia, brainstem pathology, etc.).

Clinical features

The incidence of cor pulmonale is unknown, although studies have suggested a prevalence of 0.3% in patients with chronic respiratory disease and hypoxia. Patients generally have a PaO_2 <8 kPa on air and are known to have chronic lung disease, although they may present *de novo* with cor pulmonale.

There is controversy over whether peripheral oedema and raised JVP are the result of true right heart failure or simply fluid (and salt) retention in response to renal hypoxia.

Patients may present with features of cor pulmonale during an acute exacerbation of underlying lung disease.

History

Assuming a *de novo* presentation of cor pulmonale, enquire about:

- Features of chronic lung disease. Specifically:
  - Progressive dyspnoea.
  - Smoking history.
  - Childhood respiratory disease (including asthma).
  - Sleep history (➔ Chapter 38).
  - Sputum production.
  - Previous TB (including surgical treatment).
  - Occupational history.
  - Drug history.
- Muscle weakness/swallowing difficulties.
- Fragmented sleep pattern, snoring, excessive daytime sleepiness, early morning headaches/confusion.
- Skeletal abnormalities.
- Symptoms of connective tissue disease.

Examination

Features specific to cor pulmonale.

- Signs of hypoxia (cyanosis, plethora secondary to polycythaemia).
- Signs of hypercapnia (asterixis, conjunctival redness, bounding pulse, vasodilatation, confusion).
- Raised JVP.
- Ankle/dependent oedema.
- Ascites.
- Signs of pulmonary hypertension (right ventricular heave, loud P2).
- Signs of tricuspid regurgitation (pansystolic murmur, V waves in the JVP) caused by dilatation of the RV (functional TR).

Also assess for features of possible causes (see individual chapters) as follows.

- Hyperinflation/wheeze (obstructive airways disease).
- Crackles/clubbing/poor expansion (fibrosis/restriction).
- Thoracic cage abnormalities (including surgery).
- Diaphragm weakness (abdominal indrawing on inspiration).

- Evidence of myopathy.
- Neck size.
- Evidence of connective tissue disease.

Investigations

The aim is to establish the cause of cor pulmonale.

- Pulse oximetry: cor pulmonale is unlikely if SaO_2 >92%.
- ECG: evidence of right heart strain (P pulmonale, right axis deviation, right bundle branch block).
- FBC: polycythaemia common in chronic hypoxaemia.
- ABGs: expect hypoxia and hypercapnia.
- CXR: bulky pulmonary arteries, changes consistent with underlying lung disease.
- Pulmonary function tests: obstruction/restriction.
- Echocardiography: RV structure and function, presence of tricuspid regurgitation, estimation of PAP (only if TR present).
- Overnight oximetry or sleep study.
- Nerve conduction studies/EMG.
- Tests for specific conditions (e.g. acetylcholine receptor antibodies in myasthenia) or MRI of brain.

Management

1. Treat underlying disorder

Optimise management of the underlying disease (e.g. bronchodilators, steroid therapy, CPAP).

2. Supplemental oxygen

Reversing alveolar hypoxia may prevent further increases in PAP. Caution is needed as many patients are hypercapnic, and a careful assessment is required to ensure that patients do not 'retain' CO_2 on oxygen therapy (i.e. loss of hypoxic drive). Long-term oxygen therapy (>15 hours/day) is generally required, extrapolating from two trials in COPD demonstrating improved survival on oxygen therapy.

3. Non-invasive ventilation

Long-term overnight CPAP or NIV is useful in cases of hypoventilation. Acute NIV is not required in patients with cor pulmonale unless given for acute hypercapnic and acidotic respiratory failure.

4. Diuretic therapy for peripheral oedema

Diuretics are used to prevent uncomfortable peripheral oedema. However, diuresis does not affect the underlying disease process and may exacerbate the problem (decreased filling pressure to the right ventricle). Some remaining ankle oedema is acceptable and likely, and over-use of diuretic to treat this problem is not recommended.

Prognosis

Prolonged survival (>10 years) can be seen after the first episode of peripheral oedema secondary to cor pulmonale. However, a higher level of pulmonary artery hypertension has been associated with poorer prognosis in COPD.

Chapter 9

Common chest radiograph presentations

ⓘ Unilateral lucency on the chest X-ray

Increased transradiancy of one area of the CXR or one hemithorax compared with the other. The most common cause is technical factors (e.g. rotation). This can usually be identified by comparing the degree of lucency of the soft tissues on each side.

Differential diagnosis

Pneumothorax

- Look for the thin shadow of the lung edge (visceral pleura) which should be visible in incomplete pneumothorax (➲ Chapter 55).
- Look for complete absence of lung markings lateral to this.
- Blunting of the costophrenic angle is commonly present (small associated pleural effusion).
- Complete pneumothorax: look for mediastinal shift away from the affected side.
- If mediastinal shift is marked (especially if hemidiaphragm is depressed) consider tension pneumothorax (➲ Chapter 27).
- Tension pneumothorax should be diagnosed clinically and treated immediately without a CXR.

Lung hyper-expansion

Causes

- Previous lobectomy.
- Ipsilateral collapse.
- Asymmetrical emphysema.
- Air trapping secondary to foreign body.

Bullae

These are abnormally dilated air spaces within the lung as a result of emphysematous change, usually occurring in the upper lobes. Although usually small, they may occupy one-third of a hemithorax. Their importance is that they may be mistaken for a pneumothorax in an acutely dyspnoeic patient with COPD. The round rim of a bullus may be visible and faint lung markings may differentiate them from pneumothorax. Thoracic CT is often required to be certain and should be considered if suspicious.

Chest wall abnormality

Decrease in the tissues overlying the lung may result in increased trans-radiancy. The most common cause is mastectomy, but it may also occur with congenital absence of pectoralis major (Poland's syndrome).

Pulmonary embolus

Uncommonly pulmonary embolus may be associated with oligaemic vascular markings in the affected area of the lung (Westermark's sign).

Approach to the patient

History

- Sudden onset SOB (pneumothorax, rarely PE).
- Acute chest pain (pneumothorax, PE).
- A history of COPD or long-term smoking (emphysema, bullae).
- A history of foreign body inhalation.

- Previous surgery (lobectomy, mastectomy).
- Weight loss, haemoptysis, bone pain (obstructing bronchial carcinoma, collapse).
- Symptoms of chronic infection (TB lymphadenopathy).

Examination

- Tracheal shift (pneumothorax, collapse).
- Hyper-resonant percussion + absent/decreased breath sounds (pneumothorax, bulla).
- Above + unwell patient (hypotension, profound tracheal shift): consider tension pneumothorax.
- Surgical scars (thoracotomy, mastectomy).
- Signs of obstructive lung disease (pneumothorax, bulla).
- Cachexia, lymphadenopathy (malignancy, TB).
- Check for expansion of the contralateral lung: if this is reduced, suggests this is the abnormal lung (i.e. the lung that appears lucent is in fact normal whilst the 'normal' lung has increased shadowing).

Investigations

Guided by likely diagnosis on the basis of the above.

Key points

- In tension pneumothorax, no investigations (not even a CXR) should be conducted until tension has been relieved definitively (intercostal drain placement).
- Differentiation of pneumothorax and bullae in an acutely breathless COPD patient can be difficult: thoracic CT scan is the investigation of choice.
- Lung collapse may be subtle and missed on a CXR: thoracic CT is reliable here.
- Bronchoscopy may be required to diagnose + treat foreign body inhalation.

Management

Dependent on diagnosis.

Key points

- Tension pneumothorax requires immediate treatment.
- If there is diagnostic difficulty between pneumothorax and bullae, delay drain insertion until thoracic CT imaging or senior review.
- Drain insertion into a bulla can cause substantial bleeding and result in air leak which may be resistant to treatment.
- ➲ Chapter 27 (*pneumothorax algorithm*).

ⓘ Unilateral shadowing on the chest X-ray

Unilateral shadowing on the CXR is a common clinical scenario with a wide differential diagnosis. The important features required to reach a diagnosis are as follows.

- Thorough history and examination.
- Knowledge of the differential diagnosis.
- Ability to recognise radiological patterns.
- Rapid appropriate investigations.

Abnormalities on the CXR may be chronic, and the provision of previous imaging is invaluable to assess whether the changes are new.

Differential diagnosis

Consolidation

Also known as air-space shadowing. It is caused by opacification of air spaces within the lung. Any process which results in filling (usually by fluid) of the alveoli and small airways will result in consolidation. Most patients with consolidation will be breathless and may be hypoxic (V/Q mismatch in consolidated lung).

Radiological appearance

- Ill-defined shadowing with obscured vascular markings.
- Air bronchograms are pathognomonic (air-filled bronchi contrasting against fluid-filled underlying lung).
- Usually sharply demarcated if adjacent to the pleural or interlobar fissures (➲ Chapter 55).

The differential diagnosis is wide, and only relevant acute causes are covered here.

Common

- Infection (bacterial, viral).
- Infarction.
- Cardiogenic pulmonary oedema (usually bilateral).
- Non-cardiogenic pulmonary oedema (usually bilateral).

Less common

- Drug reactions.
- Haemorrhage.
- Malignancy (lymphoma, bronchoalveolar cell carcinoma).
- Cryptogenic organising pneumonia.
- Sarcoidosis.

Pleural effusion

Fluid accumulation between the visceral and parietal pleura. ➲ Chapter 25 for causes and details on investigation.

Radiological appearance

- Around 200 ml of fluid needs to be present before visible on a PA CXR. Initially blunting of costophrenic angle (➲ Chapter 55).
- Normal appearance is of opacity obscuring hemidiaphragm with presence of a meniscus.

- If massive, may cause 'lung white-out': look for mediastinal shift away from effusion.
- Diffuse hazy shadowing throughout hemithorax in supine films.

Collapse

Partial or complete volume loss from a lung or lobe, also called atelectasis. May occur in areas of a single lobe, multiple lobes, or an entire lung.

Radiological appearance

Look for:

- Volume loss.
- Displaced fissure.
- Loss of aeration.
- Crowded bronchi/vessels.
- Compensation for volume loss.
- Elevated hemi-diaphragm.
- Displaced hilum/trachea.
- Rib crowding.
- Hyperinflation of non-involved lung.

Differential diagnosis

- Bronchial tumour.
- Enlarged lymph nodes (malignancy, TB, sarcoid).
- Viscid secretions (includes infection, post-anaesthesia).
- Pulmonary embolus (plate like atelectasis).
- Diaphragmatic weakness/paralysis (lower atelectasis).

Infarction

A rare result of pulmonary embolic disease, resulting in peripheral wedge-shaped opacities. Usually lower lobes.

Approach to the patient with unilateral chest X-ray shadowing

History

- Symptoms of infection (infective consolidation/effusion).
- Dyspnoea (speed of onset important).
- Chest pain (PE, pleural effusion, consolidation abutting pleura).
- Symptoms and risk factors for heart failure.
- Risk score for embolic disease.
- Systemic symptoms (malignancy, TB, sarcoid).
- Smoking history.
- Drug history.
- Occupational history (pleural disease).
- Pre-existing lung disease.
- Previous surgery (atelectasis, pneumonectomy).

Examination

- Thoracotomy scar.
- 'Classical' signs of consolidation (increased breath sounds, bronchial breathing ± crackles, increased vocal resonance, whispering pectoriloquy).
- Signs of effusion (stony dull percussion, decreased breath sounds, tracheal shift away if large, decreased vocal resonance).

- Paradoxical abdominal movement (diaphragm paralysis).
- Cachexia, lymphadenopathy (TB, malignancy).

Investigations

Vary depending on likely diagnosis.

Key points

- Thoracic CT valuable if diagnostic doubt (e.g. ?collapse/?consolidation).
- Thoracic ultrasound valuable to rapidly exclude effusion.
- Pleural aspiration should be performed using ultrasound guidance and delayed until further imaging if any diagnostic doubt or failed first attempt ('dry tap').
- Bronchoscopy may be used to diagnose cause of collapse.

Management

See individual sections for detailed management of each condition.

ⓘ Bilateral pulmonary infiltrates on the chest X-ray

Bilateral non-confluent airspace and interstitial shadowing is a frequent and often challenging clinical scenario. The cause may be obvious; however sometimes it is not and a thorough review of history, examination, investigations, and medications is needed. Considering the differential diagnoses in the immunocompetent and immunocompromised separately provides a structure to begin the initial assessment.

Causes in immunocompetent patients

- Infection.
  - Bacterial infection.
  - Tuberculous infection.
  - Viral infection including COVID-19.
  - Fungal infection, including PJP.
- Alveolar haemorrhage.
  - Granulomatosis with polyangiitis (GPA, previously known as Wegener's syndrome).
  - Microscopic polyangiitis.
  - Eosinophilic granulomatosis with polyangiitis (EGPA, previously known as Churg–Strauss syndrome).
  - Goodpasture's disease (anti-GBM disease).
- Pulmonary oedema.
- ARDS: non-cardiogenic pulmonary oedema.
- Interstitial lung disease:
  - Sarcoidosis.
  - UIP/NSIP/LIP/DIP/RBILD.
  - AIP: idiopathic ARDS.

Cryptogenic organising pneumonia (COP).

- Drug-induced lung disease, including illicit drug use.
- Eosinophilic pneumonia.
- Malignant disease.
  - Adenocarcinoma with a lepidic growth.
  - Lymphoma.
  - Lymphangitis carcinomatosis.
- Hypersensitivity pneumonitis.
- ABPA.

Causes of predominantly upper lobe infiltrates

- Sarcoidosis (and berylliosis).
- TB.
- Radiation therapy (may be unilateral).
- Hypersensitivity pneumonitis.
- Ankylosing spondylitis.

Causes in the immunocompromised patient

In modern medical practice, patients are frequently immunocompromised (➲ Chapter 13 for detailed discussion). Causes include cytotoxic chemotherapy, malignancy, immunosuppressive therapy for non-malignant conditions, or post-transplant and congenital or acquired immuno-deficiencies.

Such patients commonly present with acute respiratory symptoms. All the conditions which can occur in the immunocompetent individual can also occur in the immunocompromised. Infection remains the largest cause.

The differential diagnosis of bilateral pulmonary infiltrates in the immunocompromised includes the following.

- Infection.
  - Bacterial: different spectrum of organisms, including rare bacteria, e.g. *Nocardia*.
  - Viral: COVID-19, CMV pneumonitis, varicella.
  - Fungus: *Aspergillus*, PJP, *Candida, Cryptococcus*.
  - TB and non-tuberculous mycobacteria.
- Alveolar haemorrhage.
- Pulmonary oedema.
- ARDS: non-cardiogenic pulmonary oedema.
- TRALI: transfusion-associated acute lung injury may complicate patients requiring large blood transfusions.
- Drug-induced lung disease: many chemotherapy agents are associated with interstitial lung disease.
- Malignant disease.
  - Adenocarcinoma with a lepidic growth.
  - Lymphoma.
  - Lymphangitis carcinomatosis.
  - Post-transplant lymphoproliferative disease.
- Interstitial lung disease.
  - COP.
  - NSIP/LIP/DIP.
- Graft versus host disease.

Part 2

Specific clinical scenarios

Chapter 10

Inhalational injuries

Smoke inhalation

The approach to a patient who has suffered from significant smoke inhalation follows the basic airway, breathing, circulation concept. Remember to ask for details about the incident as other chemicals may have been inhaled in the smoke (see 'Hazardous chemicals' below).

The damage caused by smoke inhalation causes the following levels of injury.

Upper airways

- Laryngeal oedema.
- Mucosal inflammation.
- Ciliary dysfunction.

Lower airways

- Bronchospasm.
- Bronchial oedema/mucosal inflammation.
- Ciliary dysfunction.
- Reduced surfactant.
- Systemic inflammatory response.

Symptoms

- Hoarse voice.
- Difficulty breathing/breathlessness.
- Retrosternal chest pain.

Signs

Airway

Look for:

- Loss of eyebrows.
- Burnt nasal hair.
- Facial burns, particularly around the nose or mouth.
- Oropharyngeal burns.
- Carbonaceous sputum.
- Stridor.
- Laryngeal oedema.

Breathing

- Tachypnoea (RR > 24).
- Inspiratory crackles, wheeze, or stridor.
- Low oxygen saturations.

⚠ Saturations remain high in the presence of COHb (see 'Carbon monoxide poisoning' below).

Circulation

- Tachycardia.
- Hypotension may be present if there are large area burns to the skin or in the presence of ARDS.

Investigations

- CXR (may show pulmonary infiltrates).
- ABG.
- Measure COHb.

Management

- Early intubation in the presence of laryngeal oedema or airway burns. This may be a difficult intubation or require a surgical airway (➔ Chapter 40).
- If ventilated consider a 'lung protective' ventilatory strategy (permissive hypercapnia with low pressure/volume).
- High-flow oxygen.
- IV fluid replacement.
- Bronchodilators.
- Humidification and airway clearance techniques.
- Close observation for signs of ARDS.

Steroid use and prophylactic antibiotics are unlikely to be of benefit. Cilia and mucosal damage makes infection more likely.

Hazardous chemicals

Hazardous chemicals are used in manufacturing and the public may be exposed through accidental spills, explosions, and fires. In modern society, non-accidental release of hazardous chemicals can occur in situations associated with military use and acts of terrorism.

The effect of each chemical varies, depending upon its solubility, the mechanism by which it causes damage, systemic effects, and characteristics of the exposure. Highly soluble substances are less likely to reach the lung parenchyma.

Chemicals can produce direct cellular damage (e.g. alkalis and acids), mucous secretion, form oxygen free radicals which in turn cause damage (e.g. oxides of nitrogen), or stimulate parasympathetic receptors and trigger smooth muscle bronchoconstriction (inducing airway hyper-reactivity and bronchospasm).

Damage to nasal passages and oro-pharynx can cause:

- Oedema.
- Ulceration.
- Haemorrhage.

Damage to the trachea and bronchi can cause:

- Paralysis of the cilia.
- Increased mucous production.
- Mucosal oedema.
- Exudates.
- Submucosal haemorrhage.
- Formation of pseudomembranes.

This can result in:

- Bronchiolitis.
- Obliterative bronchiolitis.
- Organising pneumonia.

Damage to the alveoli and interstitium can cause:

- Epithelial necrosis.
- Sloughing.
- Formation of hyaline membranes.
- Alveolar capillary leakage leading to ARDS.

In the long term this can result in permanent interstitial fibrosis

⚠ Patients may still have chemical contamination both as a contact hazard and a vapour hazard. Proper precautions must be taken to avoid medical staff becoming casualties.

Management

- Assess for upper airway obstruction.
  - Look for stridor, drooling, tracheal tug.
  - Oedema, mucosal sloughing, haemorrhage.
  - Consider intubation/tracheostomy early.
- ABG.

- Assess for COHb.
- CXR (may be unhelpful early on).
- ECG.
- Supplemental oxygen (high levels may increase oxidative damage).
- Bronchodilators.
- Fluid replacement (avoid contributing to pulmonary oedema but essential in ARDS).
- Consider specific antidotes if nature of chemical exposure known (Table 10.1).
- Steroids and prophylactic antibiotics: efficacy not clear; some advocate their use.

Table 10.1 Chemical effects

Inhalant	Sources	Mechanism/injury	Treatment
Asphyxiants			
Hydrogen cyanide	Chemical warfare, burning polyurethane	Inhibits cytochrome oxidase activity, inhibiting ATP production	Hydroxocobalamin, sodium thiosulfate, sodium nitrite, dicobalt edentate
Hydrogen sulphide	Metallurgy, chemical manufacture, water treatment, volcanic gases	Inhibits cytochrome oxidase activity, inhibiting ATP production	Supportive
Carbon monoxide	Gas heaters, smoke inhalation, miners	Competes with O_2 for Hb binding sites	High-flow O_2, hyperbaric O_2
Irritant gases			
Phosgene, isocyanates	Chemical warfare, chemical and dye manufacture	Necrosis of tracheal to bronchiolar mucosa, oedema, haemorrhage, ARDS	Supportive
Ammonia	Agriculture, plastics, dyes	Irritation of mucous membranes, upper airway oedema and obstruction	Supportive
Chlorine	Household cleaners, textiles, sewage treatment, swimming pools	Liberates hydrogen chloride and O_2 free radicals. Pulmonary oedema, tracheobronchitis	Supportive
Sulphur dioxide	Smelting, paper and chemical manufacture	Pharyngeal and pulmonary oedema. Obliterative bronchiolitis	Supportive

(*Continued*)

Table 10.1 (*Contd.*)

Inhalant	Sources	Mechanism/injury	Treatment
Nitrogen oxides	Welders, dye manufacture, silo fillers, explosives use	Potent oxidizers ▸tissue inflammation + impair surfactant. Also causes metHb. Pneumonitis, bronchiolitis, pulmonary oedema	Supportive Systemic corticosteroids may benefit
Vesicant			
Mustard gas, Lewisite	Chemical warfare	Chemical pneumonitis, pulmonary oedema, pseudomembrane formation	Supportive Dimercaprol for Lewisite
Systemic toxins			
Nerve agents (Tabun, sarin, soman, ricin, VX)	Chemical warfare	Anticholinesterase effect against acetylcholinesterase. Causes meiosis, glandular secretion, bradycardia, AV block, fasciculation, paralysis, seizures, respiratory depression	Atropine, oximes (e.g. pralidoxime), benzodiazepines
Metals/metal compounds			
Cadmium	Fertilizers	Pneumonitis. Long-term causes emphysema	Supportive
Cobalt	Phosphate fertilizers	Wheezing, pneumonitis, asthma	Bronchodilators
Zinc	Zinc mining, steel manufacturing	Dyspnoea, flu-like illness	Supportive
Welding fumes	Welding	Airways obstruction	Bronchodilators
Beryllium	Limited industrial use	Pneumonitis, tracheitis. Chronic response is berylliosis (sarcoid-like)	Supportive

Carbon monoxide

⚠ Cyanosis does not occur with CO poisoning. Pulse oximetry gives false readings as COHb light absorption is similar to oxyhaemoglobin. Measure COHb if suspected.

Carbon monoxide has a 245 times greater affinity for haemoglobin than oxygen. It is not irreversibly bound and so high inspired O_2 concentrations will displace the CO from Hb. The half-life of COHb in air is 4 hours; with 100% O_2 it decreases to 40 minutes and with hyperbaric O_2 to 20 minutes.

Carbon monoxide poisoning is caused by incomplete combustion. Poorly maintained gas fires, self-poisoning, and being trapped in a burning building are the most common causes.

Clinical features

Acute

- Dyspnoea.
- Fatigue.
- Headaches.
- Tiredness.
- Tinnitus.
- Tachypnoea.
- Tachycardia.

If severe:

- Pulmonary oedema.
- Myocardial ischaemia.
- Arrhythmias.
- Seizures.
- Coma.

Late

- Cognitive deficits.
- Focal neurology.
- Personality change.

Investigations

- Remember that pulse oximetry and arterial PaO_2 may appear normal.
- Measure COHb (breath analyser, arterial or venous sample);
  - Normal COHb levels 1–2% in non-smokers, ~10% in heavy smokers.
  - >20% COHb (>10% in children) is significant CO poisoning.
  - >30% COHb confusion.
  - >35% COHb coma.
  - >50% COHb death.
- ECG.
- CXR.
- Cardiac monitor.

Management

- Give high-concentration (100%) O_2.
- If consciousness is impaired, intubate and ventilate.
- Consider hyperbaric O_2, particularly if COHb >20% or coma, as this displaces CO more rapidly (although it needs to be done early).
- Treat seizures.

Chapter 11

Inhaled foreign bodies

Inhaled foreign bodies

Everything from peas to bicycle tyre caps can make their way into the bronchial tree if circumstances allow! Lodging of a foreign body in the trachea is rare, and so this section only deals briefly with tracheal obstruction (➲ Chapter 40 for more details).

Relevant anatomy

The right main bronchus is more vertical than the left in relation to the trachea, and so an aspirated foreign body will usually (but not always) end up in the right bronchial tree, most commonly the bronchus intermedius (leading to the right middle and lower lobes) or the right lower lobe.

Presentation

►► *Acute airway obstruction*

- History of foreign body inhalation or choking.
- Conscious patient looking panic-stricken and pointing to mouth or throat. Ask if they are choking; they will nod.
- Silent breathing (i.e. not breathing).
- Paradoxical breathing pattern (seesaw breathing).
- Attempt back blows. Lean them forward and apply 5 blows between the shoulder blades using the heel of one hand.
- Attempt 5 abdominal thrusts. For a conscious person, position yourself behind them, placing a fist, thumb side in, just above the navel. Grab the fist tightly with your other hand and pull abruptly upward and inward to increase airway pressure behind the obstructing object and force it from the windpipe. The procedure may need to be repeated several times before the object is dislodged.
- If anaphylaxis and associated angio-oedema, give IM adrenaline 0.5–1 mg (0.5–1 ml of 1:1000).

►► If no improvement, call for an anaesthetist immediately, and possibly ENT surgeons.

- Apply oxygen at 10–15 L/min via reservoir bag if conscious.
- If unconscious inspect the mouth and remove any obvious obstruction.
- Start CPR.
- Leave well-fitting unbroken dentures in place.
- Anaesthetist to attempt intubation.
- Cricothyroidotomy may be required in desperate situations.

Non-emergency presentation

The most common situation is of acute onset of cough (more common than dyspnoea) after a clear history of aspiration or choking on a specific object.

Other symptoms include fever, haemoptysis, chest pain, wheeze, or stridor.

Much less common is the situation where the patient cannot remember aspirating and presents with a complication of chronic lobar occlusion (dyspnoea from lobar collapse, pneumonia, localised bronchiectasis, lung abscess), or simply as an incidental finding. It is not always obvious that an object has been aspirated rather than simply swallowed.

Evaluation

Plain CXR may show the offending foreign body if distinctly radio-opaque.

If complete lobar obstruction has occurred, subtle evidence of lobar/segmental collapse may be the only abnormality.

If the CXR is normal and there is a high index of suspicion, a thoracic CT should be performed.

Management

Spontaneous expectoration of an inhaled foreign body can occur, but is less likely if it has nestled into a lobar or segmental bronchus.

All inhaled foreign bodies should be removed to avoid the complications described above.

The majority of patients (with no acute respiratory distress or hypoxia) can be managed as outpatients. Refer to respiratory team for prompt bronchoscopy. Retrieval of inhaled foreign bodies by fibreoptic bronchoscopy is not always possible (biopsy forceps may not manage to grasp the object firmly, although using a Roth net may help) and so further referral for rigid bronchoscopy (almost universally performed in UK by thoracic surgeons) may be needed. Treat concomitant infection if present.

Chapter 12

Problems relating to adverse environments

ⓘ Diving

The respiratory problems related to diving are predominantly due to the pressure changes on air within the body and gas absorption, as well as additional complications of pre-existing respiratory conditions.

The pressure changes in diving are large. Each 10 m of descent represents 100 kPa (1 atm) increase in pressure. Most problems occur on ascending from depth. The exceptions are hypothermia (which can occur at any stage) and aspiration/drowning (normally caused by equipment failure, running out of 'air', or oxygen convulsions).

Barotrauma

This is the result of trapped gas in a body cavity expanding or compressing during pressure changes in diving. The sinuses, ears, and lungs are most commonly affected. Lung compression during a breath-hold dive can result in alveolar wall rupture, haemorrhage, and exudates.

During ascent, airspaces within the body expand. If ascent is rapid, this allows little time for any gas to escape the body via a normal route, resulting in an increased pressure in the gas pocket. In the ear this can rupture the tympanic membrane. In the lung this results in lung rupture with gas tracking to the mediastinum (pneumomediastinum), pulmonary vasculature (air embolism, see below), and pleural space (pneumothorax).

Symptoms of pneumomediastinum and pneumothorax

Chest (central) discomfort, dyspnoea, hoarseness (pneumomediastinum).

Treatment

- Supplemental (100%) oxygen.
- Needle decompression of a pneumothorax.
- Recompression in a hyperbaric chamber.

⚠ High probability that a pneumothorax will tension. This requires urgent needle decompression.

The risk of barotrauma is reduced by making slow ascents when diving. Conditions that predispose to barotrauma and are recognised contra-indications to diving are:

- Spontaneous pneumothorax (unless bilateral surgical treatment has been performed).
- COPD (if FEV_1 <80%).
- Lung bullae or cysts.
- CF (if there is pulmonary involvement).
- Fibrotic lung disease.
- Active TB.
- Active sarcoid.

Asthma

Patients with asthma may dive it they have allergic asthma but not if they have cold-, exercise-, or emotion-induced asthma.

Detailed guidelines are available from the British Thoracic Society (www.brit-thoracic.org.uk 'Diving Guidelines'). Essentially they can only dive if they are:

- Well controlled.

- Suffering no chest symptoms.
- Have not needed a therapeutic bronchodilator in the last 48 hours.
- Have normal spirometry.

For more information on medical conditions and diving, visit www.ukdmc.org/ (UK Sport and Diving medical Committee).

Decompression illness/Caisson disease

- As pressure increases during descent, nitrogen dissolves into blood and other tissues and fluids.
- Ascent should be slow to allow time for this nitrogen to come out of solution. If this does not occur, bubbles are formed, compromising blood flow.
- This condition is termed 'the bends', referring to pain in the limbs and joints caused by micro-infarction, or 'the chokes', occurring as a result of pulmonary circulation compromise from a large number of bubbles collecting in the pulmonary capillary bed (air embolism).
- This condition is most commonly caused by a rapid ascent or by operating outside the boundaries of dive tables which indicate a safe decompression plan for a given duration and depth of dive.

Symptoms/signs

- Fatigue.
- Malaise.
- Rash.
- Limb pains ('the bends').
- Paraesthesia or numbness.
- Paralysis.
- Chest tightness, cough, dyspnoea, ↓ blood pressure ('the chokes').

A pre-existing right-to-left shunt in the heart, or an AV shunt in the pulmonary circulation, can allow crossover of an air embolism, which leads to a paradoxical arterial embolus with neurological damage.

Management

- Oxygen (reduces arterial PN_2, accelerating reabsorption of bubbles).
- Lie on left side (thought to reduce the risk of an arterial embolism).
- Recompression in a hyperbaric chamber (in-water recompression by descending to depth is not advised as this process may take several hours and requires monitoring).

Flying

The major physiological challenges involved in flying relate to the effect of lower pressures on inspired PO_2 and the possibility of rapid pressure changes.

Cabin pressure

Commercial aircraft operate at cruising altitudes between 8000 m and 12 000 m. This is because these altitudes allow for greater fuel economy and avoid weather systems. Flying at these altitudes is not possible without supplemental oxygen and/or a pressurised environment (cabin pressure).

Most commercial aircraft maintain a cabin pressure of 75–85 kPa (equivalent to 1500–2400 m 'altitude') at a cruising altitude of 10 000 m. This is not a problem for most individuals but in those with lung disease this represents a potential problem of symptomatic hypoxia. The 'BTS Clinical Statement on Air Travel for Passengers with Respiratory Disease' sets out suggestions for decision making around people at risk of hypoxia:

- Patients with COPD and baseline SpO_2 ≥95% and either MRC score 1–2 or desaturation to no less than 84% during 6MWT or shuttle walk test (SWT), should be able to travel without in-flight oxygen. NB: separate guidance for restrictive lung pathologies.
- Otherwise, in flight oxygen at 2 L/min can be considered (or 2 L/min greater than LTOT prescription in those already receiving LTOT). Where there is a risk of hypercapnia a hypoxic challenge test may be needed.
- Where an HCT is required, aircraft conditions can be simulated on the ground by breathing 15% FiO_2 for 15 minutes, followed by an arterial or capillary blood gas (see www.brit-thoracic.org.uk for 'Air Travel Guidelines').

Airlines can supply additional oxygen for a flight given sufficient notice, although this may incur an extra charge.

Rapid depressurisation

Sudden loss of cabin pressure will result in loss of consciousness at altitudes above 6000 m. Supplemental oxygen is necessary in this event until the aircraft can descend to a lower altitude.

Pneumothorax

- The reduction in pressure involved in an ascent during a flight will result in expansion of gas trapped in a pneumothorax. This has the potential to convert a simple pneumothorax into a tension pneumothorax.
- Radiological evidence of resolution of a pneumothorax should be obtained prior to flying.
- Historically, a 6-week interval after complete resolution of a pneumothorax was advised before flying. However, revised BTS Clinical Statement on Air Travel for Passengers with Respiratory Disease in 2022, confirmed that the 6-week rule had been discarded and that a minimum delay of 1 week after full radiographic resolution is advised.

Non-essential air travel should be delayed for 4 weeks after thoracic surgery and at least 2 weeks for essential air travel.

The closed environment and long duration of flights means that airborne communicable diseases have the potential to spread. Individuals should not fly when they pose an infection risk to other travellers (e.g. active untreated TB and highly contagious viral infections).

Altitude

Increasing altitude results in a number of physiological stresses. There is falling ambient temperature and a reduction in atmospheric pressure with increased altitude. It is also responsible for a number of acute medical problems.

Physiology

Reduced pressure decreases inspired gas PaO_2 and hence reduces tissue availability of oxygen. Given that the fractional oxygen concentration remains constant (0.21), as does the saturated vapour pressure of water at body temperature (6.3 kPa), the inspired gas PaO_2 for a given barometric pressure can be calculated as follows:

$$\text{Inspired gas } PO_2 = 0.21 \times (\text{barometricpressure-}6.3) \text{ kPa}$$

Table 12.1 shows the pressures for varying altitudes and equivalent inspired PaO_2. It is clear that high altitudes result in significant hypoxia from the reduction in inspired PaO_2. Falling alveolar PO_2 results in a short-lived (<30 minutes) period of hyperventilation. This period is limited by hypocapnia (reducing respiratory drive) and hypoxic ventilatory decline. If hypoxia persists, there is a gradual increase in ventilation which can take several weeks to finally adjust. This acclimatisation will result in only a partial correction of the arterial PaO_2.

Table 12.1 The variation in inspired PO_2 with increasing altitude

Altitude		Barometric pressure (kPa)	Inspired gas PO_2 (kPa)
(m)	(ft)		
0	0	101	19.9
1200	4000	87.4	17.0
1800	6000	82.0	15.9
2400	8000	75.2	14.4
3000	10000	69.7	13.3
6000	20000	46.5	8.4
9000	30000	30.1	4.9
12000	40000	18.8	2.7

Acclimatisation

- There is a respiratory alkalosis with a compensatory metabolic acidosis.
- Erythropoietin production increases after a few hours to drive increased red cell production which can result in polycythaemia.
- 2,3-Diphosphoglycerate (2, 3-DPG) concentrations increase.
- There is a left shift in the oxygen dissociation curve, increasing oxygen uptake in the lungs at the expense of release to the tissues.

Adaptation

Long-term residents at high altitude have the following developmental changes.

- A blunted ventilatory response to hypoxia and exercise.
- An increased pulmonary diffusion capacity.
- Increased vascularity of cardiac and striated muscle.

Acute medical problems

The problems caused by altitude range from mild symptoms (headaches, fatigue) to life-threatening symptoms (loss of consciousness, cerebral oedema, pulmonary oedema).

Acute hypoxia

Signs/symptoms

- Impaired night vision.
- Reduced mental performance.
- Dyspnoea.
- Loss of consciousness.

Acute mountain sickness (AMS)

Occurs at altitudes >2000 m.

Signs/symptoms

- Headache.
- Dyspnoea.
- Disturbed sleep.
- Fatigue.
- Nausea.
- Poor appetite.

High-altitude pulmonary oedema (HAPE)

- Occurs at altitudes >3000 m in susceptible individuals with an exaggerated increase in pulmonary artery pressure.
- The presentation is that of classical pulmonary oedema (dyspnoea, hypoxia, cough producing pink frothy sputum, and patchy CXR changes).
- Without treatment this carries a high mortality.

High-altitude cerebral oedema (HACE)

Although this is not a respiratory problem, both HACE and HAPE can present in the same patient. Alterations in cerebral blood flow result in cerebral oedema, intracranial thrombosis, and haemorrhage.

Early signs

- Irritability.
- Ataxia.
- Irrational behaviour.

Late signs

- Hallucinations.
- Drowsiness.
- Coma.

⚠ Both HAPE and HACE are life-threatening.
Treatment involves the following.

- Supplemental oxygen.
- Reduce altitude quickly (or use a pressurised chamber).
- For HAPE: nifedipine 20 mg bd (10 mg sublingual loading dose).
- For HACE: dexamethasone 4 mg qds (10 mg loading dose).

Acclimatisation reduces the likelihood of developing AMS, HACE, and HAPE. This is achieved by a slow controlled ascent. Most of the symptoms of AMS will resolve in a few days at the same altitude.

Acetazolamide can be used to accelerate the acclimatisation process prior to the onset of symptoms or once mild symptoms of AMS develop. Nifedipine can be used as prophylaxis for HAPE, particularly if an individual has previously been affected. It does not remove the need for a controlled ascent to reduce the risks.

Sleep disturbance

At altitudes >3000 m some individuals demonstrate a periodic breathing pattern during sleep. Given the low oxygen tension already present, this gives rise to profound hypoxaemia and sleep disturbance.

Chapter 13

The immunocompromised patient

The immunocompromised patient

Acute and severe respiratory disease is more common in the immunocompromised population. Immunosuppression occurs when a person has a weak immune response which predisposes them to infection or disease. Immunosuppression can occur as part of an underlying disease process, or as a consequence of giving drugs that suppress the body's normal immune response. Drugs used include cytotoxic chemotherapy agents, corticosteroids, disease-modifying drugs, and biologic agents such as immunotherapy. Patient groups at particularly high risk are recipients of organ transplants, patients with haematological malignancies (lymphoproliferative or myeloproliferative) and those with congenital or acquired immunodeficiencies (HIV, asplenia, complement deficiency).

Certain chronic conditions (e.g. chronic lung disease, chronic liver disease, diabetes, renal failure, active malignancy, severe depression, severe frailty, old age, long-term hospital or ITU admission) can contribute to a degree of immunosuppression compared to people without the condition and should not be overlooked as contributing factors to risk of infection during clinical assessment. For a more detailed discussion see the *Oxford Handbook of Respiratory Medicine* (OHRM), Chapters 12 and 13.

Infection in the immunocompromised can be caused by common community organisms (e.g. bacteria—*streptococcus pneumoniae*, viruses—influenza), or less common organisms that most immune-competent individuals are able to protect themselves from.

Frequent or prolonged hospital admissions will expose people to hospital-acquired organisms (*Pseudomonas aeruginosa, Klebsiella pneumoniae, Staphylococcus aureus*) and drug-resistant organisms (MRSA, ESBL, CPE).

Some infecting pathogens are almost uniquely diagnosed in the presence of significant immunosuppression and often referred to as opportunistic organisms (PJP, CMV). Opportunistic infections (OIs) are a significant cause of morbidity and mortality in the severely immunocompromised.

Important considerations

- The majority (75%) of acute respiratory presentations in the immunocompromised are related to infection.
- Common community-acquired infections will still be the most likely to occur, but with increased frequency and severity.
- Suspect the possibility of atypical or opportunistic infection if the presentation or course of illness does not fit the 'classical' picture and if there has been no improvement despite adequate first-line treatment.
- 'Atypical' respiratory organisms present with symptoms such as dry cough, dyspnoea, fevers, and sweats, often with hypoxia and sometimes chest pain, weight loss, and fatigue.
- Clinical features of infection may be less pronounced in an immune-compromised host (e.g. may remain normo- or hypothermic) and there may be fewer signs and symptoms localising to the respiratory system.
- Radiological features may be more subtle.
- Non-infectious causes of acute respiratory illness include pulmonary oedema, pulmonary embolism, diffuse alveolar haemorrhage, ARDS, drug- or radiation-induced pneumonitis, post-transplant lymphoproliferative disease, graft versus host disease in stem cell transplant, and direct involvement of the underlying disease.

This discussion will focus on early assessment and treatment of emergencies, as later management should be under the guidance of the patient's main team (e.g. transplant team, HIV consultant, infectious diseases (TB), oncologist, haematologist etc.) and a respiratory physician.

ⓘ Clinical assessment

History

Features from the history may point to the underlying aetiology and help to guide management.

Timing of symptom onset in relation to the initial insult

- Acute (hours to a few days): bacterial or viral pneumonia, aspiration pneumonia, pulmonary oedema (inflammatory or left atrial hypertension), pulmonary haemorrhage, PE, ARDS.
- Subacute (days to 1–2 weeks): incomplete treatment of primary bacterial infections, secondary bacterial infections, fungi (e.g. *Pneumocystis, Aspergillus*), other bacteria (e.g. *Nocardia*, *Legionella*), viruses (e.g. CMV), idiopathic or drug-induced pneumonitis.
- Chronic (weeks to months) may indicate malignancy, tuberculous and non-tuberculous mycobacteria, fungi.
- Radiation pneumonitis typically develops 4–8 weeks after radiotherapy; immunotherapy-related pneumonitis is most common within the first 3 months of treatment.

Risks associated with types of immunological deficit

- Neutrophil abnormalities (cytotoxics, leukaemia, aplastic anaemia): bacteria, fungi.
- T-cell abnormalities (cytotoxics, post-transplant, HIV, high-dose steroids, lymphoma): fungi, viruses especially CMV, mycobacteria, *Pneumocystis*.
- B-cell or immunoglobulin abnormalities (asplenia, myeloma, lymphocytic leukaemia, lymphoma, HIV): encapsulated bacteria (*Streptococcus pneumoniae*, *Haemophilus influenzae, Neisseria meningitidis*).

Duration and severity of the immunological defect

- Mild (e.g. recurrent courses or long-term low-dose steroids, >6 months after transplantation): increased risk of infection with common community-acquired organisms (*S.pneumoniae, H.influenzae, Staphylococcus aureus,* influenza, RSV). Low risk of most opportunistic infections.
- Moderate (e.g. 1–6 months after transplantation, solid-organ malignancies receiving cytotoxic chemotherapy): common community-acquired organisms, increased risk of opportunistic pathogens.
- Severe (e.g. <1 month after transplantation; CD4<200, long-term ITU admission, advanced chronic disease; cytotoxic chemotherapy for haematological malignancies): high-risk of infection with opportunistic pathogens (CMV, *Pneumocystis jiroveci*, *Listeria, Nocardia,* mycobacteria, fungi such as *Aspergillus, Cryptococcus,* and endemic mycoses); prophylaxis often given for the most common opportunistic organisms (PJP, HSV, aspergillosis, screening for latent TB).

In general, when the immune-deficit is drug-related, dose and duration of treatment are important contributors to risk, with longer or life-long immunosuppression carrying the highest risk. In contrast, a one-off or infrequent short course of low- to moderate-dose steroids is not likely to impair the immune response.

Severity of immunosuppression may be different depending on the drug or drug combination used.

Immunosuppression related to a disease process is likely to be more significant in advanced disease (e.g. CD4 count with HIV; physiologic impairment associated with severe chronic lung disease).

Organ transplantation

The level of immunosuppression and infection risk seen in this group of patients can be stratified by organ (solid-organ vs. haematological), time since transplant (high-intensity immunosuppression necessary to prevent organ rejection in the first few days and weeks after transplantation versus long-term maintenance); and the individual risk factors associated with the donor and recipient.

HIV

- Decreased cellular and humoral immunity.
- Anyone presenting with severe respiratory infection should be offered an HIV test.
- People who are known to be HIV-positive should have a CD4 count checked on admission and early involvement of a HIV/GUM specialist.
- TB remains the leading cause of death for people living with HIV globally.
- Risk of drug–drug interactions with anti-retrovirals (ARVs) including antibiotics, which could impact efficacy of ARV therapy and/or management of infection.
- Risk of severe and/or opportunistic infection is correlated with CD4 count.
    - CD4 <200 (high-risk of infection with and death from opportunistic organisms).
    - CD4 200–500 (moderate risk, OI possible but much less likely).
    - CD4 >500 (considered 'normal', low risk).
- Immune-reconstitution inflammatory syndrome (IRIS) is a hyperinflammatory response which can occur in the first 6 months of ARV treatment for HIV as the immune system recovers which can complicate the management of opportunistic infections.
    - ARV initiation is often delayed until the person is established on OI treatment and the approach may be slightly different depending on the OI.
    - Steroids are often used in the management of moderate–severe IRIS.
    - ARV treatment should never be initiated without the guidance of an HIV specialist (GUM/ID).
- Guidelines recommend prophylaxis for certain opportunistic organisms at lower CD4 counts (<200) including PJP and screening for latent TB +/- TB preventative therapy.
- Metabolic syndrome is common in chronic HIV contributing to higher cardiovascular risk occurring at younger ages than commonly seen in HIV-negative individuals. This risk is higher if there are other concurrent CVD risk factors such as ethnicity, smoking, family history, hypertension, hypercholesterolaemia.
- Lifetime risk of any malignancy is higher compared to non-HIV infected individuals, including lung cancer. The most common malignancies associated with HIV are lymphoma (non-Hodgkin), cervical, and anal.

Examination and investigation

- ABC approach to assessment: airway management with adjuncts and ITU support if necessary.
- Check SaO_2 and ABGs as hypoxia is often worse than suspected.
- Monitor pulse, blood pressure, respiratory rate, respiratory effort. Assess fluid status.
- CXR may show focal consolidation, diffuse infiltrates, or nodularity. Comparison to previous chest imaging may be useful. CT may help if CXR non-diagnostic.
- Haemoptysis may complicate pulmonary infection or indicate an underlying neoplastic, thrombotic, or vasculitic process.
- Check FBC, U&Es, LFT, amylase, CRP, blood cultures, serology or antigen tests (e.g. CMV, HSV, RSV, urinary *Legionella* antigen), CD4 count if HIV-positive.
- FBC may show neutrophilia, neutropenia, or lymphopenia.
- Viral throat swab: influenza, COVID-19.
- All people presenting with severe pneumonia or severe sepsis should be offered an HIV test
- If risk factors are present for invasive fungal infection, consider early discussion with an infection specialist/microbiologist.
- Unless there is a strong indication, serum fungal antigen tests (e.g. Beta-D-Glucan, Galactomannan) should not form part of initial investigations as patient factors can influence test sensitivity making interpretation difficult. If a patient is considered at high risk of invasive fungal infection, empirical IV antifungal treatment should be considered and discussion with an infection specialist/microbiologist is advised.
- Check levels of immunosuppressants if relevant (cyclosporin, tacrolimus).
- Sputum should be sent for cultures requesting an atypical infection screen including fungal and mycobacterial.
- BAL samples for PCP PCR are recommended if concerned for PCP (severe immunosuppression); if bronchoscopy is not possible, induced sputum or tracheal aspirates can be used.
- Urine antigen tests for *legionella* and pneumococcus.

Management

- Supportive care with fluid balance, oxygen (keep SaO_2 >95%) and ventilatory requirements must be met. Consultation with ITU should occur early if the patient is very unwell, hypoxic with high oxygen requirements, tiring, or rapidly deteriorating and likely to require ventilatory support.
- Do not withdraw or adjust immunosuppressants without discussion with the relevant team.
- Investigate and treat pulmonary oedema and pulmonary embolus if indicated clinically.
- Commence immediate broad-spectrum antibiotic cover for any patient with neutropenia or if too unwell to wait for a definitive diagnosis. Antibiotic choice should be based on local guidelines and ideally be guided by a person's previous relevant microbiology results. 'Broad-spectrum' should include antibiotic drugs offering cover for a wide range of Gram-positive and Gram-negative +/- resistant organisms (e.g. MRSA).
- Anti-fungals (e.g. fluconazole, voriconazole; caspafungin) are not generally started as part of acute management unless there is a clear indication or on the advice of an infection specialist.
- Consider early discussion with an infection specialist/microbiologist for guidance on investigations and management. Diagnosis can be more challenging if microbiological investigations are sent after establishment on broad-spectrum treatment.
- Ideally, TB, PJP, CMV or fungal treatment should only be started after the diagnosis has been confirmed but are sometimes started empirically based on a high index of suspicion if the patient is too unwell to wait.

Role of steroids

The role of steroids in the management of acute respiratory infection remains unclear and in general, steroids are not recommended with the exception of confirmed COVID-19 infection associated with hypoxia/new oxygen requirement.

Steroids can form part of the approach to underlying non-infective respiratory pathophysiology such as exacerbations of asthma and COPD, vasculitis, immunotherapy-related pneumonitis.

Vaccination

The suppressed immune response can impact the efficacy of some vaccinations rendering them less or not effective and thus providing insufficient protection. For some vaccinations, more frequent 'boosters' can be given to elicit or maintain an immunoprotective response.

Live vaccinations are often contraindicated in the context of immunosuppression.

Vaccinations for some respiratory pathogens are recommended for people who are immunosuppressed (influenza, COVID-19, pneumococcal).

Further reading

BHIVA/BASHH/BIA Adult HIV testing guidelines, UK, 2020.

Chapter 14

Post lung transplant

ⓘ Common treatment points

This discussion will focus on diagnosis and treatment of emergencies, as later management will be based on consultation with transplant and respiratory teams. For more information see the *Oxford Handbook of Respiratory Medicine* (OHRM) Chapter 56.

- Patients may have undergone single lung transplant, bilateral sequential lung transplant, or heart–lung transplant, and would usually be discharged about 1 month after surgery.
- Common immunosuppressants used: ciclosporin, sirolimus, tacrolimus, mycophenolate, azathioprine, prednisolone.
- Ciliary function, cough reflex, blood supply, and lymphatic drainage are abnormal in the transplanted lung, predisposing to infection and injury, but oxygenation should be normal by the time of discharge. Donor lung has no bronchial circulation and relies on pulmonary vessels.
- Risk of death and of emergency complications is greatest in year one.
- Survival is 85% at 1 month, 75% at 1 year, 60% at 3 years.
- Discussion with the transplant centre should occur immediately.

Clinical assessment

- Assessment and management are broadly the same as described in the immunosuppression section; early diagnosis is often very difficult. Infection versus rejection is usually diagnosed later on bronchoscopy.
- Include spirometry at the earliest opportunity, as this will inform discussion with the transplant team. FEV_1, FVC, and TLCO rise during the first 3 months. Decline is non-specific (it may indicate airway or parenchymal disease) but is helpful to assess severity and response to treatment.
- Measure levels of ciclosporin, sirolimus, or tacrolimus.
- Before prescribing, check for interactions with immunosuppressants.

Complications

Complications within 1 month

Immediate post-operative complications

These, in general, will have been dealt with before discharge but some may very rarely present on-call. Discussion with the transplant team is essential before treating. Problems include the following:

- Re-implantation injury (usually remits by day 10), early graft dysfunction, hyperacute rejection, anastomotic breakdown, wound infection, haemorrhage, wound dehiscence, phrenic nerve injury, pulmonary artery compression/stenosis.
- Pulmonary emboli: assess and treat in the usual way.
- Pneumothorax: may occur as a surgical complication or due to invasive procedures. Treat as for secondary pneumothorax (➔ Chapter 27—pneumothorax algorithm).
- Pleural effusion: most commonly benign due to smaller size of donor lung. Usually treated conservatively. If symptoms indicate (respiratory compromise, circulatory compromise, or sepsis), perform pleural aspiration with measurement of protein, LDH, glucose levels, and pH using blood gas syringe (unless fluid purulent or contains debris). Send aspirate in blood culture bottles and plain tube for MC&S. If bloodstained, send some in an EDTA blood tube for FBC. Haemothorax is indicated by fluid haematocrit >50% of blood haematocrit. May occur as a complication of surgery or invasive procedures. Ensure adequate circulating volume and insert chest drain. Chylothorax is indicated by milky fluid with high triglycerides (>1.24 mM) and low cholesterol. May occur due to damage of the thoracic duct in surgery. Drain only if causing significant distress. Pus, pH <7.2, low glucose, or high LDH may indicate pleural infection, for which drainage and broad-spectrum antibiotics will be needed.

Graft versus host disease

Infection

- See notes on immunosuppression.
- Bacterial infection occurs in up to 35%, and is commonly due to Gram-negative organisms (e.g. *Pseudomonas aeruginosa*, *Enterobacter* spp).
- Viral pneumonia occurs in 10%.

Pulmonary oedema

- Correct fluid balance if due to volume overload.
- May be due to increased permeability or inflammatory injury.

Acute rejection

- Occurs in ~50% of patients in the first year. Usually within the first 3 months, after which other causes of dyspnoea are more likely.

- May be silent in 15–20% of patients, but usually presents with fever, malaise, cough, dyspnoea, hypoxia, and CXR infiltrates (often perihilar and lower lobe shadows with septal lines and pleural fluid).
- Most reliable sign is a fall in FEV_1 >10%.
- Discuss with transplant team. Treatment is usually 3 days of high-dose methylprednisolone after transbronchial biopsies.

Anastomotic stenosis

- Occurs weeks or months after transplant
- Causes wheeze, recurrent infection, reduction in spirometry.
- Diagnosed with CT or bronchoscopy.

Complications after 1 month

Infection

- See notes on immunosuppression (➔ Chapter 13).
- Gram-negative organisms are still more common. Therefore, if known or suspected, cover with oral ciprofloxacin or IV third-generation cephalosporin plus an aminoglycoside.
- Opportunistic infection occurs in 35–60% of patients, but may not affect mortality. CMV is the most common.
- Colonisation with *Aspergillus* is common, but active infection is rare. May cause anastomotic infection, pneumonia, bronchitis with airway pseudomembrane formation and ulceration, or disseminated disease.
- Risk of viral pneumonia continues undiminished.

Chronic rejection (or bronchiolitis obliterans syndrome)

- Progressive airway obstruction and bronchiectasis (probably due to repeated injury from microaspiration, chronic rejection, and microorganisms) causing exertional wheeze, fatigue and dyspnoea.
- Peak incidence in first 2 years, but prevalence increases with time (60–80% affected by 5–10 years).
- May present with recurrent acute bronchitis. Treat with bronchodilators, maintain oxygenation, check ABG if ventilatory insufficiency suspected (e.g. if SaO_2 <93%). Give antibiotics as for acute exacerbation of COPD, but see note above about Gram-negative organisms.

Cryptogenic organising pneumonia (COP)

- Up to 10% develop COP as part of chronic rejection.
- Presents with fever, cough, hypoxia, and peripheral consolidation.
- Treat with steroids (e.g. prednisolone 40 mg/day) and taper over months.

Post-transplant lymphoproliferative disease

- Peak incidence within first year. Affects 4–10%.
- B-cell proliferation often affects the transplanted lungs (lymphadenopathy, pulmonary infiltrates, or pulmonary nodules) and may cause peripheral lymphadenopathy, tonsillar enlargement, or skin

nodules. Often associated with EBV infection. Treated with aciclovir and reduced immunosuppression.

- T-cell proliferation may occur later and has poorer prognosis.

Renal impairment due to immunosuppressants

Recurrence

Recurrence of the disease which necessitated the transplant may occur, but rarely causes acute illness.

Chapter 15

Superior vena cava obstruction

ⓘ Introduction

Direct invasion of the SVC or compression of the vessel wall by right upper lobe tumours and/or mediastinal lymphadenopathy is the most common mechanism by which this syndrome can arise. Thrombosis within the SVC (which can occur together with direct invasion) is less common.

The cause in >90% is lung cancer (SCLC more commonly than NSCLC; present at diagnosis in 10% SCLC and 1.7% NSCLC) or lymphoma (more frequently NHL). Other rarer causes include mediastinal spread from other primary cancers (e.g. breast), thymoma, and germ cell tumours of the mediastinum. Rarer non-malignant causes include fibrosing mediastinitis.

Presentation

- Dyspnoea
- Headache
- Facial plethora
- Venous distension in the neck and distended veins on the upper chest and arms
- Upper limb oedema
- Symptoms from the primary cause may be present to varying degrees

Evaluation

In the absence of respiratory compromise (e.g. stridor from associated large airway compression) steps to establish a precise tissue diagnosis should be taken prior to starting treatment. High-dose steroids (for which there are no data confirming effectiveness) can cause dramatic shrinkage of mediastinal lymph nodes in lymphoma, making subsequent biopsy technically difficult, along with altering histological appearance of biopsies hampering diagnostic precision. Similar problems exist in establishing a precise diagnosis after radiotherapy.

CXR

May show mediastinal widening and may demonstrate evidence of an underlying lung primary.

CT scan

All patients with SVCO should have a contrast-enhanced CT scan of chest and upper abdomen as a minimum (ideally include the neck and lower abdomen/pelvis for suspected lymphoma). This will clarify a clinical diagnosis of SVCO along with providing information as to the likely underlying cause and extent of disease.

Tissue diagnosis

CT thorax may show a relatively straightforward site for obtaining histology/cytology (pleural fluid, supraclavicular lymphadenopathy, bronchoscopy if there is also suspected endobronchial disease) but ultimately mediastinal lymph nodes or tumour mass may be the only potential biopsy site. Approach may be possible under CT guidance or with endobronchial ultrasound-guided transbronchial needle aspiration (EBUS-TBNA). However, mediastinoscopy by a thoracic surgeon may be needed in a small number of cases.

Establishing a complete diagnosis in lymphoma requires good tissue samples, if requesting EBUS-TBNA for diagnosis of suspected lymphoma please specify on the request to ensure the practitioner is aware large/more samples are required if possible.

Management

In patients presenting with SVCO de novo, admission to establish a precise diagnosis is usually warranted before initiating any treatment.

Known diagnosis of lung cancer

Start steroids (dexamethasone 8 mg bd) and arrange CT thorax. Refer to respiratory/oncology team looking after the patient for consideration of SVC stenting and/or palliative radiotherapy depending on CT appearances. Prompt outpatient management is often adequate.

Palliative radiotherapy ± chemotherapy is often the first-line approach to management of SVCO caused by lung cancer. In SCLC, prompt chemotherapy without radiotherapy may be adequate.

Intraluminal stenting can be used as a primary treatment in NSCLC and may provide more rapid relief of symptoms than radiotherapy. In SCLC chemotherapy is usually the first-line treatment. Stenting is particularly important in recurrent SVCO where further oncological treatment may not be possible or successful.

Known diagnosis of lymphoma

Discuss with the haematology/oncology team looking after the patient in the first instance before commencing steroid treatment. Systemic chemotherapy (with or without radiotherapy) is the treatment of choice. The role of intraluminal stenting in lymphoma is more controversial.

Chapter 16

End-stage pulmonary disease

The WHO defines palliative care as the active total care of patients whose disease is not responsive to curative treatment. The goal of palliative care is achievement of best quality of life for patients and their families. It includes control of pain and other physical symptoms as well as care of psychological, social, and spiritual problems.

Within respiratory medicine, patients with lung malignancy are the group most often considered for palliative support, but many other patients with progressive respiratory disease (e.g. COPD, interstitial lung disease, bronchiectasis, and CF) will also benefit. In addition to specific medical therapies for symptoms, a multidisciplinary approach to offer practical support and anxiety management is indicated.

Symptoms for palliation

Pain

- Assess fully as to cause of pain.
- Treat initially with simple oral analgesia, incrementing treatment according to the WHO three analgesic stepladder (non-opioid analgesia, then weak opioids, then strong opioids) until adequate pain control.
- Prescribe adequate doses of analgesia and titrate dose accordingly.
- Ensure patient has analgesia for breakthrough pain.
- Think about alternative routes if unable to take oral medication.
- Treat side effects such as constipation and nausea effectively.
- Think about adjuvant analgesics for specific types of pain (Table 16.1).
- Consider referral to pain clinic for further interventions such as nerve blocks and transcutaneous electrical nerve stimulation (TENS).

Dyspnoea

- Breathlessness is a common symptom and is exacerbated by pain and anxiety.
- Opioids (e.g. oral morphine sulfate 2.5–5 mg) are very effective at relieving the sensation of dyspnoea without affecting respiratory function.
- If breathlessness seems disproportionate to level of underlying disease, or abruptly deteriorates, consider other possible causes (see Box 16.1).
- Short burst oxygen is often beneficial.

Table 16.1 Common adjuvant analgesics for cancer pain

Drug	Indication
Non-steroidal anti-inflammatory drugs	Bone pain Soft tissue infiltration Hepatomegaly
Corticosteroids	Raised intracranial pressure Soft tissue infiltration Nerve compression Hepatomegaly
Antidepressants (e.g. amitriptyline) Anticonvulsants (e.g. gabapentin)	Nerve compression Paraneoplastic neuropathies
Bisphosphonates	Bone pain

Box 16.1 Causes of breathlessness in lung cancer and their treatment

Lung tumour	Radiotherapy or chemotherapy
Bronchospasm	Bronchodilators
Infection	Antibiotics
Pleural effusion	Pleural drain and pleurodesis, indwelling pleural catheter
Anaemia	Blood transfusion
Pulmonary emboli	Anticoagulation
Lymphangitis	Corticosteroids
Upper airway obstruction	Stent, endobronchial Cryotherapy
SVCO	SVC stent
Pericardial effusion	Pericardial drain

Other symptoms

Cough

- Very common and can be debilitating.
- Look for reversible causes such as infection or bronchospasm and treat accordingly.
- If no reversible cause found try simple or codeine linctus. If cough persists, oral codeine or opiates act as cough suppressants and may be of benefit.
- Diazepam can also be used as a central cough depressant, especially if associated anxiety.

Anxiety

- Causes dyspnoea which worsens anxiety (leading to vicious circle).
- Benzodiazepines (e.g. lorazepam 1–4 mg sublingually) often useful.
- Midazolam best for acute panic; given IV initially 2–2.5 mg then incremental doses of 1 mg.
- Antidepressants (e.g. amitriptyline and SSRIs) are useful anxiolytics.
- Complementary therapies may be helpful (e.g. aromatherapy, hypnosis, massage, relaxation techniques).

Haemoptysis (➲ Chapter 6)

- Can be extremely frightening and occasionally catastrophic.
- Palliative radiotherapy may be useful.
- Oral anti-fibrinolytics such as tranexamic acid may help.
- Bronchial artery embolisation via interventional radiology can be considered

Superior vena cava obstruction (➲ Chapter 15)

- Presents with facial swelling.
- Diagnosis confirmed using thoracic CT with contrast.
- Start on high-dose dexamethasone (e.g. 8 mg bd) with PPI cover.
- If thrombus is present consider anticoagulation.
- Chemotherapy can be used if it is a chemo-sensitive cancer.
- Refer to interventional radiologist for insertion of SVC stent.

Poor appetite

- Common symptom due to anorexia or mouth problems, nausea, hypercalcaemia, drugs, or depression.
- May be improved in the short term by a course of oral steroids, such as prednisolone 10 mg od for 4 weeks.
- Consider nutritional supplements.

Chapter 17

Post thoracic surgery

Successful post-operative management of the thoracic surgical patient requires careful monitoring and assessment. Potential complications should be recognised and managed early, as this will reduce post-operative morbidity and mortality. Early communication with the surgical team is paramount.

Post-operative mortality and morbidity

- 30-day mortality following elective lobectomy is 1–3%, and 90-day mortality 2–6%. Minor morbidity ranges from 10–45%.
- For pneumonectomy, 30-day mortality is 6–8%, 90-day mortality 9–10%. Minor morbidity is 35–75%.
- Mortality can be up to 20% in extended pulmonary resection involving chest wall and pericardium.
- The most common complications following lung resection are pneumonia, cardiac arrhythmias, and prolonged air leak.

Respiratory complications

Respiratory problems are the most common cause of post-operative morbidity and mortality. Respiratory failure occurs in up to 2% of patients following thoracic surgery.

Pneumonia

- Common organisms: *aureus, S. pneumoniae, H. influenzae, P. aeruginosa, Klebsiella spp., E. coli, Acinetobacter spp*.
- Patients present with fever, dyspnoea, and chest pain.
- CXR may show patchy consolidation.
- Management: oxygen supplementation, antibiotics, analgesia, and chest physiotherapy.
- In severe cases, respiratory support may be required. As there is often concomitant atelectasis, NIV may be tried before invasive ventilation.

Atelectasis

- Results from the collapse of a pulmonary segment or lobe, causing hypoxia due to V/Q mismatch.
- Occurs within 24–48 hours post-operatively.
- Risk factors for developing atelectasis: poorly controlled pain, poor cough effort, and sputum retention.
- CXR typically shows volume loss ipsilaterally, mediastinal shift towards the side of the collapse, and silhouetting of the diaphragm or heart borders.
- Prevention is better than cure: Regular physiotherapy, mobilisation, incentive spirometry, breathing exercises.
- Non-invasive treatments include: physiotherapy, nebulisers, and humidified oxygen. If non-invasive measures fail to improve the situation, invasive techniques such as nasotracheal suction, CPAP, and flexible bronchoscopy for airway clearance can be utilised.

Pulmonary embolism

- Commonly occurs 10–14 days after operation.
- Presents classically with hypoxia, dyspnoea, and pleuritic chest pain.
- In the post-operative setting, it can be difficult to differentiate clinically from pneumonia.
- Confirm diagnosis with CTPA.
- Treat with anticoagulation.

Prolonged airleak

- Air leak >7 days post-operatively.
- Occurs in approximately 10% of patients after lobectomy.
- Risk factors: COPD, incomplete fissure, re-operation, decortication, lung volume reduction surgery, adhesions, incomplete lung expansion.
- Most will heal with time; conversion to a flutter bag will aid patient mobilisation.
- Consider adjunct such as blood or talc pleurodesis in selected cases.
- Re-operation and closure of the parenchymal source of the air leak is rarely required.

Lobar torsion

- Rare complication following a lobectomy; most commonly affects the middle lobe rotating around its hilar structures.
- Causes obstruction of venous return, resulting in haemorrhage and necrosis of the affected lobe.
- Occurs within 48 hours of operation but can develop up to 7 days afterwards.
- Presents with fever and haemoptysis, often rapidly deteriorating clinical condition with signs of sepsis.
- High index of suspicion is required: Serial CXRs show an increase in parenchymal opacification. CT or bronchoscopy may show a twisted bronchus.
- If torsion is suspected, the only treatment is re-operation.
- Lobar resection is required if torsion is confirmed.

Bronchopleural fistula

- Direct connection between pleural cavity and bronchial tree.
- Occurs in approximately 1–2% of patients following lobectomy and 6–10% following pneumonectomy.
- Early BPF occurs within 2 weeks after surgery, and is more common on the right, as a single bronchial artery supplies the bronchial system as opposed to two arteries on the left.
- Presents with productive cough of serosanguinous fluid, which is often positional and is caused by pleural fluid draining via the BPF into the tracheo-bronchial tree.
- Other signs: new onset fever, surgical emphysema, or increasing air leak, if the chest drain is still *in situ*.
- CXR may show an increased air space and incomplete expansion of the lung after lobectomy, or a falling air-fluid level after pneumonectomy.
- Protecting the remaining lung and confirming the diagnosis are paramount.
- Management: Chest drain into the affected side, bronchoscopy for confirming diagnosis and bronchial toileting, IV antibiotics, and nutritional and respiratory support.
- Surgery is not always required.
- Late BPF develops more than 2 months after pneumonectomy. It is usually associated with empyema and partial stump breakdown. The mortality is lower compared to early BPF.
- Management of a late BPF includes: drainage of the pleural cavity, antibiotic therapy, and nutritional support. The primary aim is to sterilise the pleural space. In some cases, the defect will heal without surgical intervention. Surgery may be considered depending on the fitness of the patient; if closure of the BPF cannot be achieved, then a permanent thoracostomy window can be created (Claggett procedure).

Post-pneumonectomy syndrome

- Mediastinal shift towards the side of the pneumonectomy, causing rotation of the heart. It causes herniation and hyperexpansion of the lung and compression of the airway.

- Rare complication which can occur months to years after pneumonectomy. The incidence is higher in young adults and children.
- Symptoms include dyspnoea, stridor, difficulty clearing secretions, episodes of acute respiratory distress.
- CXR shows extreme shifting of the heart and mediastinum into the affected hemithorax. CT and bronchoscopy can be used to identify the exact point of airway compromise.
- In severe cases, re-exploration with re-positioning of the mediastinum and filling of the pneumonectomy space is the mainstay of treatment.

Cardiac complications

- Atrial fibrillation and atrial flutter are the most common cardiac complications following thoracic surgery. They occur in 10–15% of patients after lobectomy and in 40% of patients after pneumonectomy.
- Cardiac arrhythmias are associated with increased morbidity and length of hospital stay.
- Risk factors include patient age >70, pneumonectomy, intrapericardial dissection, existing hypertension, or ischaemic heart disease.
- Treatments aim to achieve rate and/or rhythm control. Correct abnormal serum electrolytes and hypoxia. First-line pharmacological agents are beta-blockers or digoxin.
- DC cardioversion is performed if the patient is haemodynamically compromised.
- Heart failure can be caused by excessive fluid administration and right ventricular dysfunction immediately after pneumonectomy.
- The Revised Cardiac Risk Index is a tool that can be utilised to identify patients at high risk of cardiac complications following thoracic surgery.

Other complications

Surgical emphysema

- Surgical emphysema develops when air leaks under the dermal layer of the skin. It is rarely life-threatening, but often causes patient distress and increased length of hospital stay.
- Affects up to 6% of patients undergoing thoracic surgery.
- Investigations: CXR or CT chest to check whether the lung is fully expanded and if chest drain (if present) is effective.
- If the emphysema is not expanding, then conservative management is often sufficient.
- If the emphysema is worsening and the patient is distressed, a small subclavicular skin incision can be made and a negative pressure dressing applied to aid the evacuation of subcutaneous air.
- If the lung is not fully expanded, an intercostal drain should be sited. Negative pressure may be applied.
- Surgical repair of the underlying parenchymal defect may be considered in some cases.

Wound complications

- Wound infections are rare in thoracotomy wounds but are more common at chest drain sites, even after removal of the drain. Wound infections are usually limited to superficial tissue planes and are treated with antibiotics.
- Wound dehiscence requires surgical assessment and is managed by debridement and layered closure of the wound.
- Wound haematomas result from bleeding at the incision. They may worsen once low-molecular weight heparin or anticoagulants are started post-operatively. The majority improve without intervention, but large collections may become infected, and drainage may be required.
- Seromas develop due to plasma and lymphatic fluid leaking into a dead space at the incision site. Their appearance can mimic a dehisced wound with pleural fluid draining into the chest wall. Small seromas usually resolve without intervention, larger seromas can be aspirated.
- Lung herniation is caused by lung protruding through the intercostal space and occurs more commonly after minimally invasive procedures as compared to thoracotomy incisions. Patients may present with pain, swelling, and visible protrusion on coughing. Strangulation of the lung parenchyma is rare. The patient should be assessed for consideration of surgical repair.

Chronic pain

- Up to 50% of patients develop chronic pain following thoracic surgery, 25% suffer from chronic neuropathic pain.
- Risk factors for chronic pain: thoracotomy and length of surgery.
- Acute pain management: locoregional techniques such as paravertebral or erector spinae plane blocks in combination with systemic analgesia such as PCA (patient-controlled analgesia) or oral analgesics.
- Well-controlled post-operative pain reduces the rate of respiratory complications.

Assessment of the unwell surgical patient

- Follow a systematic approach for the immediate assessment, such as ABCDE.
- ABG and CXR are often requested as part of the primary assessment.
- Review available charts and clinical information, especially the operation note, and any specific post-operative instructions.
- Further imaging depends on the working diagnosis
- Early liaison with the surgical team can aid in requesting correct imaging and guiding further management.

Part 3

Acute respiratory conditions

Chapter 18

Anaphylaxis

Anaphylactic reactions (type I hypersensitivity reaction) are the consequence of the cascade caused by an IgE-mediated response to a specific antigen. Prior exposure to the antigen sensitises the individual, so that subsequent exposure results in prostaglandin-, leukotriene-, and platelet-activating factor generation and thereby histamine release. This results in vasodilatation, bronchial mucosal oedema, and bronchoconstriction.

A number of antigens can be responsible for anaphylaxis. Common causes are foodstuffs (peanuts, eggs), latex, bee/wasp stings, blood products, and drugs (vaccinations, aspirin, penicillin).

Features

- Erythema/urticaria.
- Facial/oropharyngeal mucosal oedema.
- Stridor.
- Wheeze.
- Tachypnoea.
- Warm peripheries/peripheral vasodilatation.
- Hypotension.
- Tachycardia.

Treatment

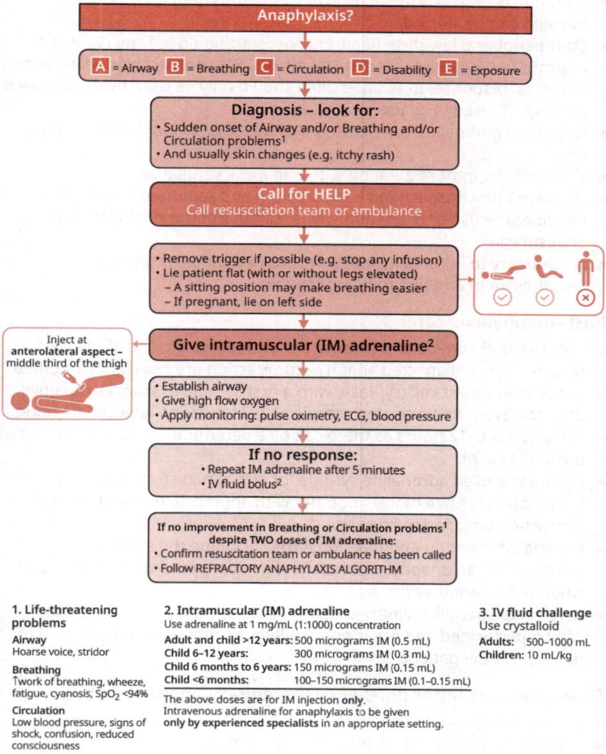

Fig. 18.1 Current anaphylaxis guidelines. Reproduced with kind permission from the Resuscitation Council.

Refractory anaphylaxis

- No improvement despite two doses of IM adrenaline. Ensure to seek expert help.
- Continue ABC approach.
- Secure airway if there are signs of airway compromise. Cricothyroidotomy may be required if airway swelling makes intubation impossible.
- Give an IV fluid bolus and titrate to response.

- Establish dedicated IV or IO access. Do not 'piggy-back' an existing IV line or use the same side as the BP cuff.
- Continue giving IM adrenaline every 5 minutes until an adrenaline infusion can be started.
- Start peripheral low dose IV adrenaline, starting dose 1 mg (1 ml of 1 mg/mL [1:1000]) adrenaline in 100 mL of 0.9% sodium chloride, titrating to clinical response. ⚠ IV adrenaline should only be used by those skilled and experienced in its use.
- Nebulised adrenaline can be used if evidence of stridor (5 ml of 1 mg/ml).
- If apneoic support respiration with bag mask ventilation.
- If severe bronchospasm give ipratropium and salbutamol nebulisers. Consider the use of IV aminophylline, salbutamol, and inhalational anaesthesia.
- If refractory to adrenaline infusion consider adding a second vasopressor in addition to IV adrenaline.

Post-anaphylaxis care

- Ensure the circumstances prior to the event, timings, and all clinical features of the suspected anaphylactic reaction are clearly documented.
- Check blood mast cell tryptase, with a first sample as soon as possible after the event and a second sample at 1–2 hours (no later than 4 hours).
- Observe for 6–12 hours as there can be a deterioration some hours after the initial event.
- Offer a pre-filled adrenaline syringe for self-administration (with a prescription for two more), together with appropriate education and instruction on using the device.
- Provide information about anaphylaxis, including the signs and symptoms of an anaphylactic reaction, avoiding potential triggers, and what to do if another occurs.
- Referral to specialist allergy centres, where specific allergen testing can be performed and occasionally allergen immunotherapy is used to desensitise the patient.

C1-esterase inhibitor deficiency (hereditary angio-oedema)

- Autosomal dominant condition.
- Ask about similar crises in other family members.
- Can be mistaken for anaphylaxis.
- Symptoms and signs primarily caused by oedema, including gastrointestinal oedema.
- Check C1-esterase inhibitor and complement levels.

Treatment

- Similar to anaphylaxis.
- Administer C1-esterase inhibitor plasma concentrate 1000–1500 units (Berinert®, Cinryze®, conestat alfa—not to be used in those with rabbit allergy), or bradykinin B2 receptor antagonist (icatibant) if available.
- If the above are not available use fresh frozen plasma (2 units).
- Unlikely to respond to antihistamines.

Chapter 19

Acute respiratory distress syndrome

Acute respiratory distress syndrome (ARDS) is a spectrum of diffuse, inflammatory lung injury that can result from a wide range of insults, most commonly pneumonia. It manifests as acute respiratory failure due to persistent lung inflammation, increased vascular permeability and reduced lung compliance. Initially described in 1967, its definition has evolved with time and certain terms such as 'acute lung injury (ALI)' have become historical. Current practice defines ARDS in accordance with the 2012 Berlin definition which requires the presence of four criteria in addition to the application of at least 5 cmH_20 of positive end-expiratory pressure (PEEP).

Berlin Definition—Criteria required to diagnose acute respiratory distress syndrome

- Onset <1 week of known insult or new/worsening respiratory symptoms.
- Bilateral lung opacities/infiltrates on chest imaging (CXR or CT).
- Pulmonary oedema not fully explained by cardiac failure or fluid overload. Consider ECHO to exclude hydrostatic pulmonary oedema.
- Hypoxaemia—PaO_2/FiO_2 (P/F) ratio <300 mmHg (40kPa).

Severity is determined by P/F ratio:

- Mild ARDS = P/F 200–300 mmHg (27–40 kPa).
- Moderate ARDS = P/F 100–200 mmHg (13–27 kPa).
- Severe ARDS = P/F <100 mmHg (13 kPa).

Recent European society of intensive care medicine (ESICM) guidelines advocate the inclusion of patients receiving high-flow nasal oxygen (HFNO) despite not meeting the PEEP eligibility criteria.

Pathophysiology

An initial insult either direct (pulmonary) or indirect (extra-pulmonary) (see Table 19.1) stimulates the release of pro-inflammatory mediators and the recruitment of neutrophils to the lungs. Subsequent damage to the alveolar capillary membrane increases its permeability causing pulmonary interstitial oedema. Translocation of interstitial fluid into the alveolar space along with neutrophils further damages the pulmonary epithelium, creating an exudate within the alveoli which in turn reduces surfactant production and promotes hyaline membrane formation. This acute exudative phase results in alveolar collapse with the loss of gas exchange surface area and reduced lung compliance. In combination with the development of pulmonary hypertension this generates large A-a gradients and significant ventilation-perfusion (V/Q) mismatching.

The following proliferative phase is dominated by micro-thrombus formation within the pulmonary vasculature, early collagen deposition, and a proliferation of fibroblasts. Rapid fibroproliferation may restore surfactant production and gas exchange but extensive damage to the alveolar membrane may lead to the third phase of widespread lung fibrosis.

Symptoms and signs

Any relating to the cause for ARDS plus:

- Tachypnoea.
- Hypoxia.
- Rapidly escalating oxygen requirements.
- Tachycardia.
- Agitation, lethargy.
- Coarse inspiratory crackles.
- CXR shows pulmonary infiltrates in an alveolar pattern. This can be patchy or unilateral initially. There may also be air bronchograms. Later stages show the more typical 'white-out'.

Table 19.1 Causes of ARDS

Direct	Indirect
Pneumonia	Sepsis
Smoke/toxic inhalation	Massive trauma
Gastric aspiration	Transfusion of blood products
Near drowning	Burns
Lung contusion	Acute pancreatitis
Amniotic fluid embolus	Cardiopulmonary bypass
Fat emboli	Eclampsia
	DIC
	DKA
	Drugs, e.g. opiates, aspirin
	Head injury/raised ICP

Management

Treat the underlying cause of ARDS. Avoid further lung injury and provide best supportive care.

- ABG assessment of hypoxaemia and PCO_2 (low initially but hypercapnia develops as respiratory failure worsens).
- Current evidence recommends the consideration of HFNO and/or CPAP (5–10 cmH_2O) to reduce the risk of intubation but this may only be temporary.
- Intubation and ventilation according to the ARDSnet trial using lung protective ventilation (LPV). Including tidal volumes of 6 ml/kg, plateau pressures <30 cmH_2O, and permissive hypercapnia.
- The use of proning is strongly recommended in those with moderate to severe ARDS given the significant reduction in mortality demonstrated in the PROSEVA trial.
- The use of higher PEEP is recommended in patients with moderate ARDS with subsequent neuromuscular blockade (NMB) recommended in those progressing to severe ARDS.
- Guidelines strongly recommend against the use of recruitment manoeuvres and high frequency oscillatory ventilation (HFOV).
- Systemic corticosteroids are now recommended for all patients with ARDS following the findings of the DEXA-ARDS trial and the COVID-19 specific RECOVERY trial.
- CVP monitoring is favoured over invasive cardiac monitoring such as pulmonary artery catheters.
- Conservative fluid balance targets are recommended given the risk of worsening pulmonary oedema.
- CVP monitoring is favoured over invasive cardiac monitoring such as pulmonary artery (PA) catheters, which are associated with higher rates of complications.
- Inotropic support and renal replacement therapy are frequently required as ARDS commonly results in multi-organ failure.
- Enteral feeding via a NG tube is recommended.
- Culture any potential infective source (sputum/BAL, urine, blood) and consider broad-spectrum antibiotics. Inflammatory markers are likely to be raised in ARDS even in the absence of infection.
- Patients with severe ARDS and a high Murray score (3 or greater) or pH <7.20 on optimal management should be referred to the local extracorporeal membrane oxygenation (ECMO) centre.

A number of other treatments have been trialed in ARDS but there is limited evidence of a survival benefit.

- Surfactant replacement.
- Inhaled nitric oxide.
- Nebulised epoprostenol.

Prognosis

Mortality has improved over the last 20 years because of improvements in supportive care and ventilator strategies. Mortality in severe ARDS however remains approximately 45%. Increasing age, multi-organ failure, and a direct pulmonary cause of ARDS are poor prognostic markers. Over half of survivors will have a degree of residual lung damage and a reduced functional capacity as a result.

Resources

Qadir N et al. An update on management of adult patients with acute respiratory distress syndrome. Am J Respir Crit Care Med 2024; 209: 24–36. https://doi.org/10.1164/rccm.202311-2011st

Grasselli G et al. ESICM guidelines on acute respiratory distress syndrome: definition, phenotyping and respiratory support strategies. ICM 2023; 49: 727–759. https://doi.org/10.1007/s00134-023-07050-7

Chapter 20

Asthma

Definition

'Asthma is a heterogeneous disease, usually characterized by chronic airway inflammation. It is defined by the history of respiratory symptoms, such as wheeze, shortness of breath, chest tightness and cough, that vary over time and in intensity, together with variable expiratory airflow limitation' (GINA 2024: www.ginasthma.org).

The prevalence of asthma is increasing, more so in children than adults, with an estimated 300 million people with asthma and approximately 250,000 deaths per year. The highest levels of asthma are seen in developed countries. It is the most common chronic respiratory condition in the UK with a prevalence of 12%.

In the UK there are peaks of asthma deaths, in the summer in younger patients and in the winter in older patients.

Symptoms and signs

Symptoms

- Wheeze.
- SOB.
- Chest tightness.
- Cough.

These symptoms tend to be:

- Variable.
- Intermittent.
- Worse at night and/or early morning.
- Triggered. Common triggers include:
  - Allergens.
  - Respiratory infections.
  - Irritants.
  - Weather.
  - Exercise.
  - Medication.
  - Emotional stress.

Other features

- Family (or personal) history of asthma or atopy.
- Worsening symptoms with medication, e.g. aspirin or beta-blockers.
- Be aware of occupational asthma. Ask if symptoms are better at weekends or holidays.

Signs

- None.
- Wheeze: diffuse, polyphonic, expiratory, bilateral.
- May have reduced peak flow/FEV1 (normal between exacerbations).

Diagnosis

This is a clinical diagnosis based on a combination of symptoms and confirmatory objective measures.

Objective measurements

- ≥ 12% FEV_1 (or 200 ml) improvement after bronchodilator administration (salbutamol 200mcg MDI via spacer or 2.5 mg via nebuliser) or corticosteroid trial (14 days, 30 mg prednisolone per day).

OR

- Positive methacholine or mannitol challenge test.

OR

- Peak flow variability of >20% between highest and lowest values when taken 4x day or more for 2 weeks.

Differential diagnosis

- COPD.
- Cardiac disease.
- Tumour:
  - lung.
  - tracheal.
  - laryngeal.
- Foreign body.
- Bronchiectasis.
- Interstitial lung disease.
- PE.
- Aspiration.
- Inducible laryngeal obstruction.
- Breathing pattern disorder.

Management of acute asthma

History

- There is often a history of symptoms suggesting worsening asthma in the preceding few days.
  - Increasing use of β_2 agonist, including overnight.
  - Nocturnal cough.
  - Early morning chest tightness.
- Obtain information on background asthma control (before this attack).
  - Frequency of daily use of short-acting β_2 agonist.
  - Number of prior admissions to hospital over past year.
  - Prior admissions to ITU.
  - Best PEF if known (within last 2 years).
- Look for trigger factors.
  - Associated infection.
  - Known allergen.
  - Change in asthma medication (or run out or non-compliant), or introduction of new medication (e.g. NSAIDs or beta-blockers).

Examination

- Observations:
  - SaO_2.
  - Respiratory rate.
  - Heart rate.
  - Blood pressure.
  - Temperature.
- PEF measurement: pre-nebuliser.
- Auscultation of chest.

Investigations

- FBC.
- Theophylline level, if usually taken.
- CXR (to exclude pneumothorax and to look for infection).
- ABG if SaO_2 <92%.

Grading of severity of the acute exacerbation and subsequent management is guided by the PEF recording and examination of the patient for pulse, BP, RR, ability to complete sentences, and air entry.

- Mild: PEF ≥75% predicted.
- Moderate: PEF 50–75% predicted.
- Severe: PEF 33–50% predicted.
- Life-threatening: PEF <33% predicted.

If the patient is seen in the community (or A&E), admit if PEF <50% or there are concerns regarding ability to respond to symptoms, social concerns, exacerbation occurring late in the day, or prior history of difficult-to-treat asthma.

Those patients who are at increased risk of death from asthma include:

- Those with severe asthma.
- Known difficult-to-treat asthma or previous near fatal asthma.

- Those with severe asthma and adverse behavioural or psycho-social features, including:
  - Non-compliance, previous self-discharge.
  - Psychiatric illness.
  - Social isolation.
  - Alcohol or drug abuse.
  - Learning difficulties.
  - Obesity.

All patients with asthma should have (if required):

- High-flow oxygen, maintaining oxygen saturations 94–98% unless otherwise indicated.
- Nebulised bronchodilators driven by oxygen, or bronchodilators given via MDI and spacer.

Management algorithms

Mild exacerbation

- PEF ≥75% predicted.
- Give usual bronchodilator.
  - In mild–moderate exacerbations β2 agonist via MDI and spacer device is as effective as a nebuliser.
- Check at 15–30 minutes:
  - PEF ≥75% and clinically stable: no further treatment, observe for 2 hours and discharge if stable (see discharge planning below).
  - PEF ≤75% but clinically stable—treat as moderate exacerbation.

Algorithms for moderate exacerbation, acute severe asthma, and life-threatening asthma are shown in Figs. 20.1, 20.2, and 20.3, respectively.

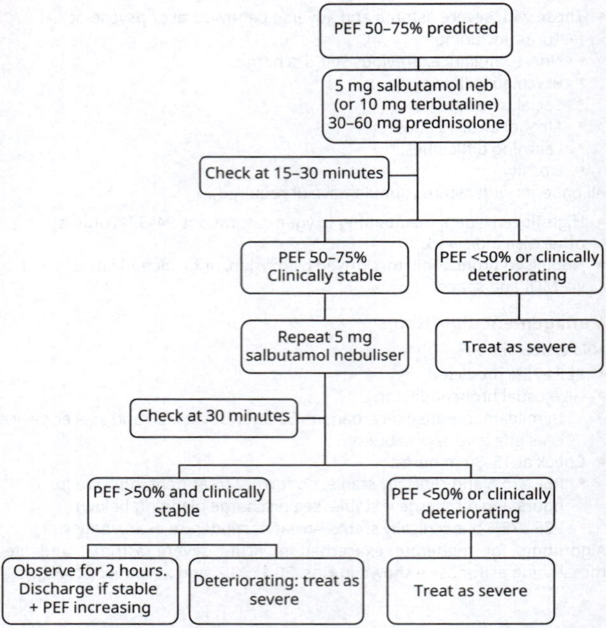

Fig. 20.1 Moderate asthma exacerbation. Algorithm from the BTS Asthma Guidelines (www.brit-thoracic.org.uk).

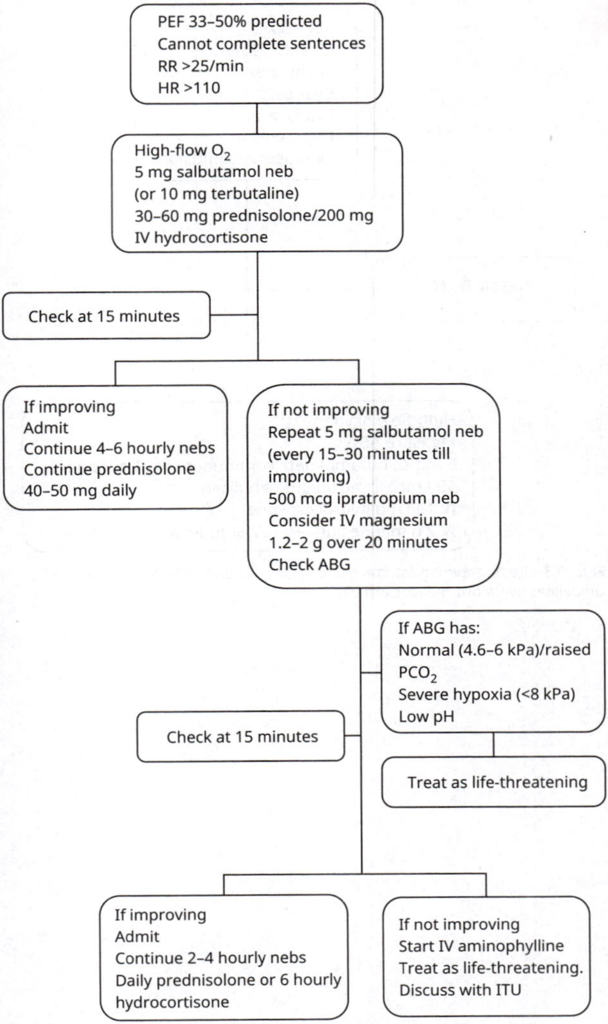

Fig. 20.2 Severe asthma exacerbation. Algorithm from the BTS Asthma Guidelines (www.brit-thoracic.org.uk).

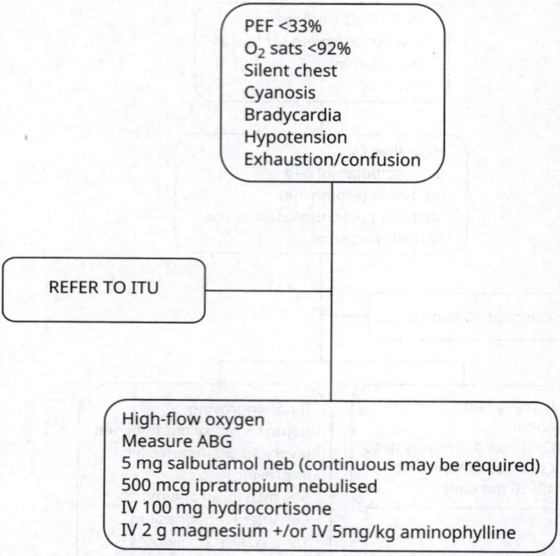

Fig. 20.3 Life-threatening asthma exacerbation. Algorithm from the BTS Asthma Guidelines (www.brit-thoracic.org.uk).

Asthma in pregnancy

- Acute asthma should be treated as per the non-pregnant patient: asthma medications are regarded as safe in pregnancy and should be continued or initiated without hesitation.
- Risk to mother and fetus are much greater from uncontrolled asthma than from its treatment.
- Maintain oxygen saturations >95% to prevent fetal hypoxia.
- Obstetric advice should be sought: continuous fetal monitoring is recommended in severe asthma. Earlier intensive care involvement may be indicated.
- ➲ Chapter 4.

Patients on asthma biologics

More recently disease-modifying biologic medications have been developed for use in those with severe asthma not controlled with standard therapies. These medications should be continued in patients admitted to hospital either with asthma exacerbations or other medical problems (exception: Tezepelumab should be held if the patient has an acute infection if a dose is due whilst the infection is ongoing).

If you are not sure whether the biologic medication should continue or be held, you should discuss this with your local respiratory team.

Discharge planning

- Patients should be on home medication for 24 hours prior to discharge (i.e. off nebulisers for 24 hours)
- PEF >75% predicted and <25% variability.

On discharge, all patients should have:

- Prednisolone 40 mg for at least 5 days.
- Oral antibiotics if confirmed evidence of infection.
- Supply of all inhalers and technique checked.
- PEF meter.
- Written self-management plan.
- Advised to see GP or asthma nurse within the next few days.
- Letter to GP re: admission.
- Those with severe asthma should be referred for follow-up in the chest or specialist asthma clinic. Repeat attendees to A&E should also be considered for referral to optimise their asthma management.

Chapter 21

Chronic obstructive pulmonary disease

Chronic obstructive pulmonary disease (COPD) is increasing in frequency worldwide, particularly in developed countries, and has a major impact in terms of mortality, morbidity, and overall healthcare burden. In 2015, approximately 3.2 million deaths were secondary to COPD, with the condition being the fourth leading cause of death globally. In the UK, it is the second largest cause of acute admissions (~130,000/year) and it accounts for 1.4 million GP consultations annually. Approximately 90% of cases of COPD are smoking-related, with the remainder being secondary to occupational and environmental exposures, genetics, and in-utero injury. Management is focused on smoking cessation, pulmonary rehabilitation, optimisation of comorbidities, inhaled therapies, and prevention of exacerbations.

Diagnosis

History and examination

The diagnosis of COPD is based on symptoms and signs (such as cough and breathlessness), and risk factors and is supported by spirometry. It should be considered in those over 35 years of age with a risk factor and one or more of the following symptoms:

- Shortness of breath on exertion.
- Chronic cough.
- Regular sputum production.
- Frequent winter 'bronchitis'.
- Wheeze.

Enquire about weight loss, ankle swelling, functional limitation, the severity of breathlessness (using the mMRC dyspnoea scale) and occupational exposures. Ask about symptoms that would point to other pathologies such as diurnal variability, a nocturnal predilection for symptoms, young age (<35 years), eczema and rhinitis (asthma), chest pain (e.g. cardiovascular), excessive sputum production, and haemoptysis (e.g. bronchiectasis).

Spirometry

Spirometry should be performed for diagnosis of COPD.

- Obstructive picture with reduced FEV_1 (<80% predicted) and FEV_1/FVC ratio <70% .
- Use standard residuals (SRs, z-scores) instead of predicted percentage cutoffs to avoid underdiagnosing younger patients and overdiagnosing older patients. -1.645 is defined as the lower limit of normal.
- Pulmonary function tests may also show raised total lung capacity and residual volume due to air trapping, and reduced gas transfer due to emphysema.

Radiology

Chest X-rays may show hyperexpanded lungs in cases of emphysema. CT chest can identify emphysema, air trapping, and coexisting conditions such as bronchiectasis.

Acute exacerbation of chronic obstructive pulmonary disease

An exacerbation is defined as an acute and sustained worsening of symptoms causing a patient to seek medical advice, beyond normal day-to-day variation. It is a clinical diagnosis based on symptoms:

- Worsening breathlessness.
- Cough.
- Increased sputum production or change in sputum colour.

Causes

Usually infective, either viral or bacterial or in combination (typically *Haemophilus influenzae*, *Streptococcus pneumoniae*, and *Moraxella catarrhalis*), but can also be secondary to pollution or another insult to the lungs.

Other differential diagnoses to consider in a patient with COPD presenting with increased shortness of breath are pneumothorax, pulmonary emboli, cardiac dysfunction, lobar or segmental collapse due to sputum retention or tumour.

Assessment of severity

A brief history should be taken to gain an idea of premorbid functional abilities, previous admissions to hospital or intensive care, level of usual treatment (home nebulisers and/or oxygen), and comorbidities.

Respiratory rate >25 and use of accessory muscles indicate respiratory distress. In addition, all patients should have their BP, heart rate, respiratory rate, temperature, and oxygen saturation (ideally on air) recorded.

After the initial assessment, a decision should be made as to where the patient is best managed (Table 21.1).

Table 21.1 Decision to treat at home or in hospital

Factor	Treat at home	Treat in hospital
SOB	Mild	Severe
General condition	Good	Poor/deteriorating
Level of activity	Good	Poor/confined to bed
Speed of onset	Gradual	Rapid
SaO_2 <90%	No	Yes
Acute confusion	Absent	Present
Conscious level	Normal	Impaired
Cyanosis	Absent	Present
Peripheral oedema	Absent	Present
Social situation	Good	Living alone, not coping
Premorbid level	Good	Poor
Significant comorbidity	No	Yes
CXR changes	No	Yes
Arterial pH	≥7.35	<7.35
Arterial PaO_2	≥7 kPa	<7 kPa

Investigations

- FBC (anaemia, infection).
- U&Es (dehydration, renal failure, watch K+).
- Theophylline level if on oral theophylline.
- Blood cultures if pyrexial.
- Sputum culture.
- CXR (to look for pneumonia and rule out pneumothorax).
- ABG (to assess pH and to guide oxygen therapy; see below).
- ECG.
- CTPA (if PE is suspected as a cause for deterioration).

Management

Oxygen ⓘ administration and target saturations should be based on ABG results (➔ Chapter 42). Whilst waiting for the results the main focus should be on correcting the hypoxia; depending on clinical suspicion, aiming for saturations of 88–92% is not unreasonable. It is not uncommon to find significant hypercapnia in a patient brought in by ambulance where uncontrolled oxygen has been given; treatment with appropriately controlled oxygen therapy often corrects this.

Nebulised bronchodilators should be administered on arrival (driven via air if there are concerns regarding type 2 respiratory failure):

- 2.5–5 mg salbutamol plus 500 mcg ipratropium bromide QDS.

Corticosteroids (oral prednisolone 30 mg/day or IV hydrocortisone 100 mg 6-hourly if too unwell to have oral medication) should be started in all patients presenting with a significant exacerbation and should be continued for 5 days, as they shorten recovery time. Longer courses increase the risk of complications (e.g. pneumonia, sepsis, and death).

Antibiotics should be given to patients who have three main symptoms:

- Increase in SOB.
- Increase in sputum volume.
- Increase in sputum purulence.

Also treat if they have two of the above but sputum purulence is one or if they require mechanical ventilation (invasive or non-invasive).

Non-invasive ventilation (NIV) (➔ Chapter 44) should be started in those patients with an acute exacerbation of COPD who fail to respond to initial maximal medical therapy and appropriate controlled oxygen therapy with:

- pH < 7.35 and
- $PCO_2 > 6$.

In most cases, NIV should be commenced at an IPAP of 10–12 mmH_2O, and an EPAP of 4–5 mmH_2O. Oxygen can be entrained to maintain SaO_2 between 88% and 92% and nebuliser treatment (via air) should be continued. Before starting NIV a clear decision should be documented as to whether this is the ceiling of treatment or whether the patient should have invasive ventilation in the event of failure of NIV. NIV is not usually indicated in those with end-stage disease and poor performance status.

IV aminophylline should only be considered in those not responding to nebulised treatment. Certain guidelines do not recommend this treatment at all due to the high risk of interactions and side effects. Those not on oral theophylline before admission should receive a loading dose followed by a maintenance infusion.

- Loading dose: 5 mg/kg given in 250 ml 5% glucose or 0.9% saline over 0.5–1 hour.
- Maintenance dose of 0.5 mg/kg/hour (diluted with 5% glucose or 0.9% saline).

Theophylline levels should be measured within 4–6 hours after starting treatment, and then daily, to guide treatment and prevent toxicity.

Early discharge schemes

Hospital-at-home and assisted-discharge schemes are now available, with studies indicating they are safe and effective. Generally, these are suitable for patients without poor prognostic factors such as acidosis. Explore what is available at your hospital.

Discharge planning

- Consider discharge once the patient is approaching their usual premorbid level of functioning.
- Ensure patients are re-established on their inhaler bronchodilator therapies and that they are using them effectively.
- If tolerated, measure spirometry in all patients before discharge.
- Assess all aspects of care, i.e. smoking cessation, vaccinations, side effects of medications, reasons for poor compliance, need for long-term oxygen, and need for long-term ventilation.
- Ensure the patient can manage at home successfully; work with the family and the MDT.
- Ensure the patients and their families have all the information they require.
- Consider referral for pulmonary rehabilitation/commence inpatient pulmonary rehabilitation if available.
- Refer to COPD community teams to increase support and prevent future admissions, and arrange early follow-up as needed.

Further reading

1. Chronic obstructive pulmonary disease in over 16s: diagnosis and management. NICE guideline [NG115]. DOI:10.3233/TAD-181100.
2. Global strategy for the diagnosis, management, and prevention of chronic obstructive pulmonary disease. GOLD report 2024. DOI:10.1016/S2213-2600(23)00461-7.

Chapter 22

Breathing pattern disorders

Breathing is a natural process and occurs with no thought. There are many reasons why breathing can lose its natural rhythm and cause the individual to experience unpleasant sensations of breathlessness disproportionate to the level of activity. Breathing pattern disorder (BPD) is defined as a chronic or recurrent condition where 'the normal biomechanical pattern of breathing is disrupted, resulting in dyspnea and associated non-respiratory symptoms that cannot be fully explained by disease pathophysiology.' These specifically relate to over breathing, ranging from simple upper chest or apical breathing to, at the end of the scale, hyperventilation.

Patients with BPD tend to breathe in a manner that is disconnected from their respiratory and metabolic requirements, and in some cases can lead to a decrease in their $PaCO_2$ through hyperventilation. BPDs are seen when individual uses the wrong muscles to breathe. BPD may be present in the absence of a respiratory condition (primary BPD), or it may accompany another respiratory condition, mostly asthma and more recently long COVID (secondary BPD).

Classification

- Hyperventilation syndrome.
- Periodic deep sighing.
- Thoracic dominant breathing.
- Forced abdominal expiration.
- Thoraco-abdominal asynchrony.

Diagnosis

Diagnosing BPDs requires a comprehensive patient history (Table 22.1), physical examination, and additional tests to rule out organic causes.

- Consider triggers and alleviating factors.
- Associated symptoms (anxiety).

Table 22.1 Commonly reported symptoms of BPD

Episodes of breathlessness usually unrelated to exercise but can be made worse by exercise or activity.
Noisy breathing both during inspiration and expiration.
Difficulty coordinating breathing, talking, and eating.
Symptoms of light-headedness or dizziness.
Pins and needles in fingertips, hands, and around the mouth.
Feeling of unsatisfied breath.
Palpitations.
Chest pain.
Headache.
Bloated feeling in the stomach.
Fatigue.

Differential diagnosis

BPD can mimic cardiac, neurological, and gastrointestinal conditions. These medical conditions must be ruled out:

- Anaemia.
- Asthma.
- Pneumonia.
- PE.
- COPD/emphysema.

Investigations

ⓘ Need to rule our organic pathology.

- U&Es and LFT.
- CXR.
- PFTs.
- ECG.
- ABG.
- A normal SaO_2 at rest and on exercise to the point of breathlessness is usually indicative of a breathing pattern disorder.
- Capnography to measure end-tidal CO_2.
- Questionnaires:
  - Nijmegen Questionnaire for hyperventilation symptoms.
  - Brompton Breathing Assessment Tool (BPAT).

Treatment approaches

Refer to a specialist in treatment of BPD, often a respiratory physiotherapist.

Breathing retraining

Breathing retraining focuses on teaching patients to learn to breathe less. Techniques include:

- Diaphragmatic breathing: Encouraging the use of the diaphragm rather than accessory muscles.
- Pursed-lip breathing: To slow down breathing and improve oxygenation.
- Controlled breathing: Techniques to reduce respiratory rate and depth.

Psychological interventions

There is a strong link between BPDs and psychological factors, therefore including mental health support is essential.
Cognitive behavioural therapy (CBT): Helps patients address and modify dysfunctional thoughts and behaviours related to breathing. Mindfulness and relaxation techniques: Meditation and progressive muscle relaxation aim to reduce overall stress and improve breathing.

Physical therapy

Physical therapy can be beneficial in addressing musculoskeletal components of BPDs.

Postural training: Exercises to correct postural abnormalities that affect breathing.

Patient education

Educating patients about their condition empowers them to take an active role in their management.

Provide information about how dysfunctional breathing patterns develop and their impact on QoL.

Advice on how to manage symptoms and prevent exacerbations. Consider altering lifestyle factors such as diet and sleep hygiene.

It takes time and practice to change a poor breathing habit, but restoring a normal breathing pattern can relieve many of the unpleasant symptoms associated with BPD.

References

1. Ionescu MF, Mani-Babu S, Degani-Costa LH, Johnson M, Paramasivan C, Sylvester K, Fuld J. Cardiopulmonary exercise testing in the assessment of dysfunctional breathing. Frontiers in Physiology. 2021 Jan 27;11:620955. https://doi.org/10.3389/fphys.2020.620955
2. Grillo L, Russell AM, Shannon H, and Lewis A. Physiotherapy assessment of breathing pattern disorder: a qualitative evaluation. BMJ Open Respiratory Research. 2023;10(1):e001395. https://doi.org/10.1136/bmjresp-2022-001395

Further reading

For further information on management of BPD refer to www.physiotherapyforbpd.org.uk

Chapter 23

Respiratory infections

Bacterial pneumonia

Pneumonia is defined as an infection of one or both lungs causing the alveoli to fill with pus and inflammatory fluid. It has classically been diagnosed based on common clinical symptoms and radiological features seen on CXR or CT imaging.

Pneumonia can be sub-classified based on the pattern of infection (lobar or bronchial), origin, mechanism, and most likely contributing organisms including bacterial, mycobacterial, viral, fungal, and other atypical organisms.

Anyone can get pneumonia, but it is more common in the following groups:

- People >65yrs.
- Young children.
- Smokers.
- Alcohol dependence.
- Chronic medical conditions putting them at increased risk (e.g. lung disease, liver disease, renal failure, heart failure, immunosuppression).

Investigations

- Observations: Oxygen saturations, respiratory rate, BP, HR.
- Bloods: FBC, UE, LFT, ABG if new oxygen requirement.
- Blood cultures if pyrexial or signs of sepsis.
- Sputum for MC&S.
  - Moderate sensitivity.
  - Quality of lower respiratory sample increases test sensitivity.
- Urine legionella and pneumococcal antigens in moderate to severe presentation.
- Respiratory viral PCR.
- CXR.

Community-acquired pneumonia (CAP)

Pneumonia identified at presentation or within 48 hours of hospital admission. Leading cause of hospitalisation and death globally. There may be a history of past or intercurrent viral infection (influenza, COVID-19).

Presentation: Cough productive of purulent sputum, fever, pleuritic chest pain, breathlessness, haemoptysis.

Common organisms: *Streptococcus pneumoniae, Haemophilus influenzae* (*Staphylococcus aureus* and some atypical organisms such as *Mycoplasma pneumoniae*).

Gram-negative bacteria and anaerobes are less common.

Staphylococcus aureus

- More common in immune-compromised hosts (e.g. haematological malignancy, alcohol dependence, drug-users, very young, and elderly).
- Can cause bilateral cavitating bronchopneumonia.
- Can be the result of haematogenous spread in someone with staph aureus bacteraemia associated with pulmonary abscesses (look out for signs of infective endocarditis).
- Can complicate influenza infection.
- The most effective treatment for confirmed meticillin sensitive *staphylococcus aureus* (MSSA) infection is flucloxacillin (vancomycin or teicoplanin if MRSA is confirmed or suspected).

Classification of severity

The CURB-65 score (Table 23.1) is a validated clinical tool for estimating the severity of CAP and indicating the need for hospital admission. The mortality risk at 30 days associated with CAP increases as the CURB-65 score increases.

Table 23.1 CURB-65 score and classification

CURB-65	
Symptom	**Points**
Confusion (AMTS </= 8)	1
Urea (>7 mmol/L)	1
Respiratory Rate (>/= 30/min)	1
Blood Pressure (<90 systolic and/or 60 mmHg diastolic)	1
Age >/=**65yrs**	1

Score	Indication for management
0-1	Outpatient management
2	Consider hospital admission
3 or above	Hospital admission advised

Other concerning features which increasing mortality risk:

- Significant comorbidity.
- Bilateral/multi-lobar involvement.
- Hypoxia with PaO_2 <8 kPa/SaO_2 <92% .

Management

- Check local antibiotic guidelines.
- Note the most common cause, *Streptococcus pneumoniae,* is usually very sensitive to penicillin/amoxicillin and other beta-lactam antibiotics and first-generation cephalosporins.
- Resistance of *Streptococcus pneumoniae* isolates to penicillin and macrolides (e.g. clarithromycin) are rare in the UK but growing (more common in the USA, Southern Europe).
- Common first-line options: monotherapy with PO/IV amoxicillin; PO clarithromycin or doxycycline if penicillin allergic.
- In unwell hospitalised patients with a documented penicillin allergy, IV treatment with vancomycin or teicoplanin is advised.
- Course length: 5 days oral treatment is usually enough for milder cases; 5–10 days in more severe cases (14 days in bronchiectasis).
- Severe hospitalised cases (CURB-65 score of 3 or above, ITU admission, oxygen requirement, significant comorbidity) may require empirical combined antibiotic therapy of a beta-lactam such as penicillin, amoxicillin or co-amoxiclav, and either clarithromycin or doxycycline until the infecting organism is identified or clinical improvement.
- Consider antibiotic doses and route of administration alongside severity.
- Radiological improvement may lag behind clinical improvement.
- The BTS recommends repeat CXR 6 weeks after treatment completion for people with persistent signs or symptoms or where there is concern

for underlying malignancy (particularly smokers and people >50yrs)—only if they would be fit for further investigation (i.e. not severely frail or comorbid patients).

- People over the age of 65yrs or those younger with significant comorbidity should be offered pneumococcal vaccination when well (once only lifetime dose).

Atypical organisms

Pneumonia caused by less common 'community-acquired' organisms. Organisms difficult to isolate in culture (intracellular) and less visible on Gram-stain. Atypically grouped organisms have similar presenting signs and symptoms. Most 'atypical' bacteria lack cell walls and therefore cannot be successfully treated with beta-lactam antibiotics.

Antibiotic options

- First-line: Macrolide (e.g. clarithromycin, azithromycin) or tetracycline (e.g. doxycycline).
- Second-line: Fluoroquinolone (levofloxacin), used with caution due to risk of significant side effects (tendonitis, tendon rupture, QT prolongation, Clostridium difficile).

*Combined beta-lactam and macrolide/tetracycline courses are often used in severe cases to ensure antibiotic cover for the most common and atypical community-acquired pneumonia.

Atypical organisms to consider

- *Legionella*—often causes systemic symptoms, confusion, and hyponatremia. Associated with contaminated and stagnant water sources (e.g. air conditioning units). Do legionella antigen test. Treat with clarithromycin or levofloxacin for 5–10 days.
- *Mycoplasma pneumoniae*—often mild and more common in school-age children. Can cause a rash and jaundice. Do a PCR on sputum for reliable results. Treat with doxycycline or clarithromycin.
- *Chlamydia pneumoniae*—often mild and does not always require antibiotic treatment.

Hospital-acquired pneumonia (HAP)

Pneumonia that develops >48 hours after hospital admission and was not felt to be incubating at the time of admission (nosocomial). Gram-negative and drug-resistant organisms more likely.

Risk factors

- Individual patient risk factors (concurrent severe acute illness, comorbidities, immunosuppression).
- Length of hospital stay.
- Staff adherence to infection control procedures.

Common organisms: Aerobic Gram-negative Enterobacteriaceae (*Klebsiella pneumoniae, Pseudomonas aeruginosa, Escherichia coli, Acinetobacter spp). Staphylococcus aureus,* inc. MRSA.

Pseudomonas aeruginosa

- Risk in those with chronic lung disease (bronchiectasis, COPD, CF).
- Associated with poorer outcomes in people with bronchiectasis, contributing to a more rapid decline in lung function.

- Once isolated in sputum, considered chronically colonised.
- Decision to cover with antibiotics active against pseudomonas should be based on frequency and timing of isolates containing pseudomonas for that individual, and tested sensitivities.
- High level of intrinsic resistance to many antibiotics.
- The choice of antibiotic should be based on individual sensitivities as there is often resistance to multiple antibiotics. There are often no oral options. Consult your local microbiologist for advice.

Treatment considerations

- Lung abscesses can be associated with pyogenic bacteria known to cause HAP (e.g. *S. aureus, Pseudomonas aeruginosa, Klebsiella pneumoniae*). Longer courses of treatment may be needed.
- Broader spectrum antibiotics with enhanced Gram-negative cover may be needed when compared to CAP.
- Consider individual risk of resistant organisms (e.g. previous MRSA infection).

Ventilator-associated pneumonia

Pneumonia that occurs 48 hours or more after endotracheal intubation. A sub-type of hospital-acquired pneumonia. Majority (over 90%) of pneumonias identified in ITU are in intubated and ventilated patients.

Culture of endotracheal aspirates and bronchoscopic samples (endotracheal aspirates have a lower yield and are more likely to be contaminated with non-pathogenic oral flora).

Common organisms: As with HAP (higher risk of resistant organisms).

Aspiration

Evidence of pneumonia or acute respiratory infection in the hours to days following a suspected or witnessed episode of aspiration. The majority of aspiration episodes result in a chemical pneumonitis, without progressing to bacterial pneumonia. Right lung more commonly affected due to the angle of the carina.

Risk factors

- Reduced level of consciousness.
- Dementia.
- Delirium.
- Seizures/post-ictal.
- Drug/alcohol intoxication.
- Neurological conditions, e.g. MND, MS, previous stroke.
- Oesophageal disease.

Treatment considerations

- Can lead to lung abscess and empyema.
- Often polymicrobial, consider usual organisms but also Gram-negative organisms from the GI tract.
- Usually single agent with amoxicillin or doxycycline is appropriate but sometimes metronidazole is added for anaerobic cover.
- Consider factors contributing to aspiration and mitigate these to prevent recurrent episodes.

Influenza and parainfluenza viruses

Human

Seasonal influenza often referred to as 'the flu' is an acute respiratory infection caused by one of the human influenza viruses common in all parts of the world. Transmission is highest during the colder months of the year.

Usually presents with:

- Fever, chills.
- Myalgia.
- Headache.
- Sore throat.
- Cough.
- Fatigue.

Non-flu viruses such as RSV, rhinoviruses, and SARS-CoV-2 can cause similar symptoms. Viral swabs may test for several of these viruses routinely.

Investigation

Viral PCR from throat swab.

Management

Consider oseltamivir if:

- Presentation within 48 hours of symptom onset.
- The person is in an 'at risk' group—e.g. elderly, frail, comorbid, pregnant, immunocompromised.
- Consider antibiotics **only** if features of secondary bacterial infection are present.

Anti-virals are not indicated in non-hospitalised uncomplicated infection.

Vaccination

- Flu vaccine efficacy is approx. 40–60% varying season on season. It is designed to reduce the severity of illness and complications, to reduce hospitalisations and death.
- Vaccination is recommended annually in autumnal months for those at risk of complications such as the elderly, very young, pregnant women, immunocompromised patients, and those with chronic disease. It is also offered to front-line health and social care workers.

Zoonotic variants

Some subtypes of influenza type A can infect animals. These subtypes are distinct from human types and are known as variant influenza viruses. Infected animals shed influenza virus in saliva, nasal secretions, and faeces. Humans most at risk of variant influenza are people in close contact with certain animals or contaminated environments. Human to human transmission of variant influenza viruses is possible but rare.

Symptoms are very similar to human strains of influenza and can range from mild to severe. Variant influenza strains should be considered in those who have exposure to infected or possibly infected animals or contact with those who are known to have variant influenza.

Strains of note

- H1N1v—'swine flu'.
    - Caused a global pandemic in 2009–2010 with estimated deaths of 151,700–575,500 worldwide.
    - H1N1v is now a seasonal circulating influenza virus in humans so is no longer referred to as swine flu.
- HPAI—highly pathogenic avian influenza—'bird flu'
    - Few avian influenza viruses have crossed the species barrier to infect humans, the most notable one being H5N1v which is highly pathogenic and has caused major outbreaks in 2019/2020 and 2023/2024.
    - There have been 900 known likely infections in 2023/2024 with a 50% mortality rate (although milder cases may be under-represented in the data).

Management

- As per human influenza strains, oseltamivir or zanamivir may be given if within 48 hours of symptom onset and confirmed positive for influenza A
- Strict isolation is recommended, with those admitted to hospital placed in negative pressure side rooms and airborne pathogen precautions being taken by staff and laboratory workers.
- If a variant influenza strain is suspected, urgent advice from the local on-call infection specialist should be sought immediately.
- The seasonal influenza vaccine does not protect against any zoonotic variants and there are no specific vaccines currently available.

Coronaviruses

Severe acute respiratory syndromes (SARS-CoV-1 and SARS-CoV-2)

SARS-CoV-1 was initially identified in Guandong province, China in November 2002 and was recognised as a global threat in February 2003. It was quickly identified as being easily spread by air travel and was a short-lived threat, causing only 8098 reported cases with 774 deaths worldwide. The last case was identified in July 2003.

SARS-CoV-2 is a genetically similar virus which led to a much larger and more widespread pandemic in 2020–2021. It was initially identified in Hubei province, China in 2019 and the ensuing pandemic was known as the COVID-19 pandemic. When compared with SARS-CoV-1, SARS-CoV-2 is much more virulent and deadly. WHO estimates that in 2020 alone, 3 million deaths worldwide could be attributed to COVID-19. It also caused widespread disruption to normal life and the economy due to strict lockdowns imposed by many nations designed to try and reduce the spread of the virus.

Although cases of COVID-19 are still present amongst the population, they are generally less deadly and far less common than seen during the 2020–2021 pandemic due to increased immunity in the population, widespread vaccination of those most vulnerable, and mutations in the virus causing different strains to be more prevalent.

SARS-CoV-2/COVID-19

- Originally an animal virus that has crossed the species barrier.
- Incubation period of 2–10 days.
- Felt to be infectious until 10 days from symptom onset or once a previously positive lateral flow test is negative.

Presentation

- Usually mild and self-limiting flu-like illness.
- Adults more likely to have serious disease—especially those with risk factors such as being older, obesity, and having comorbidities like diabetes, and chronic heart and lung disease. Some ethnicities, those living in socio-economically deprived areas, and men were also at higher risk of severe disease during the 2020–2021 pandemic.
- Severe disease presents initially with flu-like illness and progresses to respiratory symptoms and then in some cases respiratory failure requiring intensive care support in the most serious of cases.
- Mortality rate varied between 0–50% of cases during the initial pandemic, varying widely across different countries.
- Complications include:
  - Clotting abnormalities (both clots and bleeding).
  - Multi-system inflammatory syndrome—leading to acute cardiac, liver, and kidney injury.
  - Bilateral pneumonia, ARDS, and respiratory failure.
  - Chronic morbidity from persistent symptoms after viral clearance—now known as 'Long COVID'. Can cause symptoms such as fatigue, breathlessness, arthralgia, memory problems, and dizziness. Mechanisms contributing to this remain poorly understood.

Investigations

- Baseline observations.
- Routine bloods—lymphopenia might be present on FBC, CRP could also be significantly raised. U&Es and LFTs can be abnormal in more severe disease.
- Blood and sputum cultures if super-imposed bacterial infection is suspected.
- Pharyngeal throat swab for respiratory PCR—most centres now process samples for influenza A&B, RSV, and COVID-19 together.
- Urine for *Legionella* & pneumococcal antigens if bacterial pneumonia suspected.
- CXR (or CT thorax)—common early features of widespread bilateral patchy changes. Fibrosis, cystic changes, and pneumothorax can follow. CTPA should be performed if there are symptoms suggestive of PE.

Management

- Usually supportive and can be managed at home.
- In those with mild disease but at risk of deterioration, antivirals such as Paxlovid can be provided if the disease is identified early.
- In those hospitalised with severe disease requiring oxygen or mechanical/non-invasive ventilation:
  - Dexamethasone 6 mg PO/IV for 10 days or until hospital discharge.
  - Tocilizumab or baricitinib if the patient has raised inflammatory markers but no suggestion of significant concurrent bacterial infection.
  - Remdesivir IV for 3–5 days if presentation is within 10 days of symptom onset.
- Antibiotics only indicated if secondary bacterial infection is suspected or confirmed.
- For those hospitalised with severe disease, oxygen supplementation may be required and early intensive care input should be sought in those deemed suitable for mechanical ventilation or CPAP.
- Prone positioning can be considered.
- In the most severe of cases ECMO can be used although the mortality in these cases was very high.

Vaccination

- The COVID-19 vaccine was developed rapidly and the first doses were administered to the public in December 2020.
- There were some controversies around safety concerns and side effects of the vaccines given their rapid development.
- More people have now been vaccinated against COVID-19 than any other disease and the vaccines have been shown to be overwhelmingly safe and effective at reducing the severity of disease and risk of hospitalisation and death. There will always be a small number of people who suffer significant side-effects or allergy, as with any intervention.
- Repeated vaccination is required in certain populations due to constant evolution of the virus. Those populations include those over 75, those with weakened immune systems, those resident in care homes, and front-line health and social care workers.

Middle Eastern respiratory syndrome (MERS)

- MERS was first identified in Saudi Arabia in 2012 and has remained most prevalent in the Middle East since then. There have been 2622 reported cases with 953 deaths.
- Transmission is from contact with infected camels or humans.
- Most human cases present with severe respiratory disease and MERS has a 35% mortality rate.
- A MERS-CoV PCR can be done in suspected cases but only usually processed in national reference laboratories.
- Management is supportive only and there is no available vaccination.

Fungal infections of the lung

Invasive fungal lung infections are rarely seen in immunocompetent patients but can be life-threatening in those with underlying immune-compromise.

Global incidence is increasing likely due to a combination of improved reporting, better and more sensitive diagnostic testing, along with increased use of immuno-suppressant therapies.

Pneumocystis pneumonia (PCP or PJP)

- *Pneumocystis jirovecii* (PJP) is a fungal organism that can cause pneumonia in immunocompromised patients.
- Incidence in those with HIV and solid organ transplants has fallen due to widespread use of prophylaxis.
- Earlier establishment of ART after HIV diagnosis has reduced the frequency of infection in this population.

Presentation

- Dry cough, dyspnoea, exertional hypoxia, fevers, and chest pain.
- Extra-pulmonary manifestations such as: hepatomegaly, lymphadenopathy, skin lesions, retinal cotton-wool spots, thyroid masses.
- Mortality is between 10–50% depending on severity and underlying comorbidity.

Investigations

- Exertional oxygen saturation monitoring if not requiring oxygen supplementation at rest.
- Arterial blood gas to assess severity of hypoxia.
- HIV test, if HIV status not known, CD4 count if known to be HIV-positive.
- Sputum, induced sputum, or bronchoalveolar washings for culture.
- Beta-d-glucan is non-specific but could be helpful if PJP is strongly suspected.
- CXR—diffuse bilateral infiltrates are a classical sign but can appear normal.
- CT thorax—patchy ground glass opacification with interlobular septal thickening +/- cysts.

Treatment

- Empirical treatment often commenced whilst awaiting investigations, especially if the patient is unwell.
- First-line treatment is with co-trimoxazole (either oral or IV depending on severity of disease), although allergy is common and alternatives can be used.
- Prednisolone 50–80 mg PO OD should be given in cases where oxygen supplementation or ventilation is required, and a weaning course is often needed.
- Prophylaxis is often considered in those deemed at highest risk (e.g. HIV patients with CD4 count <200, solid organ transplant patients, and those having chemotherapy or bone marrow transplant for haematological malignancy) and is often with a lower dose of co-trimoxazole or alternative.

Invasive pulmonary aspergillosis (IPA)

- Caused by *aspergillus fumigatus* or *aspergillus flavus*.
- Most common in those with haematological malignancy or bone marrow transplant recipients. Can also present in critically unwell patients on the ICU.

Presentation

- Dyspnoea, cough, chest pain, fever not responding to broad spectrum antibiotics, haemoptysis.
- Can lead to ARDS and has high mortality (up to >90%).

Investigation

- Serum galactomannan.
- Serum beta-d-glucan can be useful in high-risk patients but not specific to *Aspergillus*.
- Sputum +/- bronchial wash for PCR, culture, and galactomannan.
- CXR +/- HRCT—scattered nodules with 'halo' sign, air crescent, tree-in-bud changes, bronchial wall thickening, and cavitating consolidation.

Management

- In suspected IPA, initiate anti-fungals early and then undertake investigations to confirm. Seek early microbiology input.
- First-line—voriconazole, can also use alternative triazoles.
- Second-line—amphotericin B (+/- echinocandin).
- Beware interactions with immunosuppressive agents.

Chapter 24

Tuberculosis and non-tuberculous mycobacteria

Tuberculosis

Tuberculosis (TB) remains a major global health threat. In 2022, TB was the second leading infectious disease killer after COVID-19, killing 1.3 million people, around 13% of whom were HIV-positive. Most global TB-related deaths occur in the WHO African and Southeast Asian regions. It is estimated that around a quarter of the world's population have been infected, with 5–10% of infected people developing active disease in their lifetime.

In 2022, eight countries accounted for around two-thirds of global TB cases: India, Indonesia, China, Philippines, Pakistan, Nigeria, Bangladesh, and the Democratic Republic of Congo. Incidence of TB in the UK is considered low at around 8 per 100 000 (2022 data). It is predominantly seen in large urban centres (London, Birmingham, Manchester) and most common in people born outside the UK or who spend a significant amount of time in TB-prevalent countries.

Pathophysiology

Mycobacterium tuberculosis

Mycobacterium tuberculosis (MTB) is spread via airborne droplet nuclei when people cough or sneeze. Primary infection occurs in the lungs after inhalation, though it can later spread to anywhere in the body. Infection with MTB is now considered to exist along a continuum from non-infected to clinically active; only those with 'active' pulmonary TB are considered infectious.

Non-infected: the immune system may kill the bacillus soon after inhalation.

Quiescent TB infection: the bacillus may be contained, but not cleared by the immune system and become dormant (latent), during which time the person remains asymptomatic. The bacillus may later reactivate, usually at times of immune-system stress or immunosuppression.

Incipient: prolonged asymptomatic phase of TB infection with assumed progression towards symptomatic clinically active disease. Considered non-infectious.

Subclinical active infection: oligo- or asymptomatic, non-infectious or periodically infectious.

Clinically active infection: Infectious, symptomatic infection associated with clinical, radiological, and microbiological signs.

Pulmonary tuberculosis (PTB)

History of productive cough for more than 2 weeks, sometimes with haemoptysis, associated with fever, night sweats, weight loss, and anorexia with symptoms emerging over a period of weeks to months.

It is common for people with active pulmonary TB to have a history of partial or no response to one or more antibiotic courses prescribed for suspected LRTI/CAP.

Differential diagnosis of pulmonary tuberculosis

- Bacterial pneumonia.
- Non-tuberculous mycobacterium of the lungs.
- Chronic pulmonary aspergillosis.
- Nocardia.
- Malignancy.

Investigations

History: clinical symptoms, close contacts, previous treatment for TB, country of origin, travel history, comorbidities.

Radiology: CXR or CT chest.

Haematology/biochemistry: FBC, U&E, LFTS, and CRP.

Virology: All patients with confirmed or suspected TB should be tested for HIV. Hepatitis B and C screening is not routinely recommended, though could be offered to people with associated risk factors as co-infection could have treatment and monitoring implications.

Microbiological: At least three sputum samples (preferably one sent early morning) for AFB smear and culture; blood cultures. Consider bronchoscopy and lavage if initial sputum negative and the index of suspicion for PTB remains high

Molecular tests: Reverse Transcriptase-PCR, nucleic acid amplification tests (NAAT), whole genome sequencing (WGS). Detect MTB-DNA or RNA and resistance to rifampicin. E.g. Cepheid Xpert MTB/Rif® assay, Trunat® assays.

Extrapulmonary tuberculosis (EPTB)

Though all primary infection is considered pulmonary, MTB has the capacity to spread to other areas of the body via haematogenous spread and can occur at any other body site.

Common sites

- Pleural.
- Pericardial.
- Bowel and GI-tract: Leading to abdominal pain, ascites, malabsorption.
- Adrenal.
- Genitourinary: Epididymitis in men; pyelonephritis.
- Gynaecological: Presenting commonly as pelvic inflammatory disease (PID) or fallopian tube dysfunction leading to infertility. Quite often diagnosed during investigations for underlying female infertility.
- CNS: Tuberculomas; TB meningitis: Presents with persistent headache for days to weeks ± fever, reduced or fluctuating level of consciousness or focal neurology.
- Lymph node: TB lymphadenitis. Presents with enlarged painless or painful lymph node(s) ± systemic malaise. Most common in cervical lymph nodes.
- Skeletal: Spine, long bones, joints. Usually presents with pain in the affected area (most frequently the spine but can occur anywhere), often with associated systemic upset including fever, sweats, and weight loss.
- Disseminated ('miliary'): Miliary pattern seen on CXR. More common in children and immunosuppression. Associated with a high mortality.

Investigations for extrapulmonary tuberculosis

Investigations depend on the site affected but generally should include:

- Imaging of the site (XR, US, CT, MRI).
- Microbiology: tissue samples for staining and microscopy, PCR testing, and MTB culture. Types of tissue can include a biopsy sample, pleural fluid, ascitic fluid, CSF.

- A microbiological diagnosis with antibiotic sensitivities to the core drugs (rifampicin and isoniazid) is needed for the best chance of treatment success.
- All efforts should be made to gain adequate samples for testing.
- Involvement of surgical teams (general, ENT, orthopaedics, spinal, gynaecological) may be needed depending on the site.
- A negative test result does not necessarily exclude active TB. If the index of suspicion remains high despite negative tests (or lack of samples) a decision about empirical treatment will need to be made based on risk factors and the absence of a convincing alternative diagnosis.
- Rapid nucleic acid amplification tests (NAAT): include GeneXpert, TruNat.

Measures of immune response to mycobacterium tuberculosis

Tuberculin skin test (TST): Subcutaneous injection of tuberculin and the localised immune response is measured.

Interferon Gamma Release Assay (IGRA): Blood test. Useful in identifying latent TB or past exposure, but unable to differentiate between the two.

They cannot detect active disease and are not useful as part of an acute respiratory diagnostic work-up.

Treatment: Drug-sensitive

Principles of tuberculosis treatment

- Based on individual antibiotic sensitivity profile for core drugs (rifampicin, isoniazid +/- fluoroquinolones).
- Multi-drug regimens.
- Combination of drugs chosen for their action against TB bacilli.
- Dosed to reach therapeutic blood levels (considering weight, absorption/excretion, co-drugs and comorbidities).
- Duration (dependent on TB-site, host factors, individual response to treatment).
- Adherence support (DOTS, VOTS).

Standard quadruple therapy

- When MTB sensitive to both rifampicin + isoniazid, known as drug-sensitive TB (DSTB).
- Easy to remember with the acronym 'RIPE' (**R**ifampicin (R), **I**soniazid (seen as I or H), **P**yrazinamide (seen as P or Z), **E**thambutol (E)). Side effects are shown in Table 24.1
- Although in the UK this four-drug regimen is traditionally documented as HRZE.

Standard courses for PTB and EPTB are for 6-months split into the 'intensive phase' where all four drugs are given for the first 2 months followed by a 'continuation phase' of 4-months rifampicin and isoniazid alone. Cure rates are>95% with this regimen.

Shorter treatment regimens

Based on the results of several clinical trials investigating shorter, efficacious regimens for DSTB, a 4-month regimen (rifapentine (Rif), isoniazid (I or H), moxifloxacin (M), pyrazinamide (P or Z)) was found to be as effective as the 6-month RIPE regimen and can now be prescribed for people over the age of 12yrs.

Table 24.1 Common tuberculosis drugs and toxicity

Drug	Toxicity	Baseline assessment and monitoring
Rifampicin	Orange body secretions (urine, tears), GI upset (nausea, diarrhoea), hepatitis, renal failure, thrombocytopenia, significant drug interactions (CyP450 pathway)	FBC, UE, LFT, medication history
Isoniazid	Hepatitis, peripheral neuropathy*, drug-induced lupus, agranulocytosis	FBC, LFT, peripheral nerve examination
Moxifloxacin	QTc prolongation, tendon rupture	ECG
Pyrazinamide	Rash, nausea, hyperuricaemia/gout, arthralgia, hepatitis, hypothyroidism	LFT, TSH
Ethambutol	Optic neuritis	Visual acuity and colour vision assessment using Ishihara

Multi-drug-resistant tuberculosis

It is estimated that around 25% of all TB deaths are related to drug resistance. This is characterised by the presence of resistance to rifampicin or isoniazid, as the two are the most important drugs in the regimen. Drug-resistance can be *acquired* (new resistance mutations occurring spontaneously) or *transmitted* from person to person. Acquired resistance can occur if there has been poor adherence or incomplete treatment (including exposure to antibiotics active against MTB when used for other indications), treatment given at incorrect doses, due to malabsorption, or if too few TB-active drugs are used.

Multi-drug regimens protect against the development of resistance, which is more likely in the acute phase of treatment when the mycobacteria are most active. The most common form of resistant TB seen in the UK is isoniazid mono-resistance.

Risk factors for multi-drug-resistant tuberculosis include:

- Previous episodes of confirmed or suspected treated TB.
- History of suspected or confirmed TB treatment failure.
- Contact with a known case of drug-resistant TB.
- Born in or emigration from a country known to have high prevalence of MDR-TB (e.g. The Russian Federation, WHO Eastern European region, Central Asian region, India, China, Pakistan).

Treatment: Drug-resistant

Historical treatment for MDR-TB required long courses (12–24 months) of five to seven medications (oral and injectable), leading to challenging and often irreversible side effects. Recent drug developments mean an effective, well-tolerated, 6-month, all oral regimen is now possible for the majority of people with MDR-TB, irrelevant of HIV status.

The WHO 2022 guidelines recommends a 6-month BPaLM regimen (bedaquiline, pretomanid, linezolid, moxifloxacin) for eligible people with rifampicin-resistant TB. Further information can be found in *the Oxford Handbook of Respiratory Medicine*, chapter 43.

Monitoring response to treatment

Patients should be assessed at baseline before starting treatment and at specified time intervals during and at the end of treatment using a combination of the following:

- Clinical symptoms
- Radiology
- Microbiological (sputum smear and/or culture)

HIV and tuberculosis

TB is the leading cause of death amongst people living with HIV (PLWH), who are at greater risk of contracting TB and of developing more severe forms of TB infection. The risk of contracting TB and its manifestations is related to the host immune response indicated by CD4 count. Presentation will likely be 'typical' if the CD4 count >500 cells/μL. Increasingly lower CD4 counts infer a greater risk of 'atypical' presentation.

Investigation considerations:

- PLWH are more likely to have smear negative sputum.
- Consider bronchoscopy if suspicion remains despite negative samples.
- Consider investigation results carefully alongside the history, symptoms and presentation, risk factors for contracting TB (CD4 count, known positive contact, time spent in areas of high TB prevalence).
- WHO guidelines recommend using more sensitive NAATs such as *XPert Ultra*, able to detect MTB at lower thresholds.
- Lateral flow urine lipoarabinomannan assay (U-LAM/ TB-LAM) is a point of care test for detecting mycobacterial lipoarabinomannan antigen in HIV-positive patients with a low CD4 count (sensitivity reduced at CD4 counts >200 cells/μL); not suitable for HIV-negative patients due to reduced sensitivity.
- CXR changes may be atypical (miliary, less likely to develop cavities).
- Extrapulmonary forms of TB are more common.

Management of TB-HIV co-infection

Anti-tuberculous treatment is equally effective in those who are HIV-positive as in those who are HIV-negative, although the treatment raises some key issues.

Drug–drug interactions

- Protease inhibitors (PI) and non-nucleoside reverse transcriptase inhibitors (NNRTI) are metabolised via the cytochrome p-450 pathway and interfere with the metabolism of rifampicin. Their combination should be avoided.
- Involvement of a HIV specialist is essential.

Malabsorption

- Some patients with low CD4 counts may have concurrent GI opportunistic infection which can impair absorption.
- Protease inhibitors can cause diarrhoea.
- Timing of administration (around food or other medication).

Immune reconstitution inflammatory syndrome (IRIS)

- If HAART is started at the same time as TB treatment, rapid reconstitution of CD4 and the immune response initiation of HAART has been shown to produce a sustained rise in the CD4 count, leading to a restoration of immunity to the mycobacterial antigen, which in turn causes a clinical and radiological deterioration in those with TB at a median time of 12 days.
- It is recommended that, in those with HIV-TB co-infection not yet established on treatment, the start of HAART is delayed until TB treatment has been initiated which reduces the risk of IRIS.
- Usually mild and self-limiting but corticosteroids are sometimes required.

Tuberculosis in pregnancy

All pre-menopausal adult women and their partners are recommended to take measures to avoid pregnancy whilst receiving TB treatment to avoid any potential concerns associated with transmission or side effects of treatment. Re-activation of latent TB is considered more likely during pregnancy. TB presents as in non-pregnant individuals, although diagnosis may be delayed because of hesitation to do a CXR in early pregnancy.

Treatment

- **DS-TB pregnant or breast-feeding:** The standard 6-month RIPE regimen is recommended; not currently eligible for the 4-month DSTB regimen.
- **DR-TB pregnant or breast-feeding:** eligible for 6–9-month regimens containing bedaquiline and delamanid.

Treatment efficacy is the same as in non-pregnant individuals; late diagnosis increases the risk of intrauterine growth retardation, low birth weight, pre-eclampsia, stillbirth, and obstetric mortality. The risk of congenital infection or infection at delivery is extremely rare; highest for a baby born to a smear-positive mother who has had <2 weeks active treatment (in this case preventative isoniazid treatment of the neonate should be considered).

Babies felt to be at higher risk of TB (living in or regularly visiting high prevalence areas) should be BCG vaccinated at birth.

Post-tuberculosis lung disease

Post-TB lung disease (PTLB) is a chronic lung disease (CLD) caused by previously treated pulmonary TB. The focus of global TB efforts has until recently, been on improving diagnosis and access to effective treatment, meaning the evidence base for PTLD is sparse. Presentation is varied and the respiratory morbidity attributable to PTLD is correlated with the severity and number of previous episodes of active TB, timing of treatment initiation, and effectiveness of prior treatment.

The spectrum of PTLD is varied and can present as restrictive, obstructive, or mixed pathology, with similarities of presentation to other CLD such as COPD and bronchiectasis. Individual patient factors also play a role including asthma, smoking, and occupational lung disease.

Investigation considerations

- Symptoms alone are not enough to indicate recurrent TB infection.
- PTLD patients will have chronic respiratory symptoms and could be prone to developing significant respiratory symptoms during infective and non-infective exacerbations (e.g. productive cough, haemoptysis, breathlessness, hypoxia, chest pain).
- They have a higher risk of recurrent episodes of TB (reactivation or reinfection), and bacterial, viral, and fungal lung infection, when compared to people without PTLD.
- TB test interpretation is more challenging, even more so in those who are HIV-negative. Sputum PCR tests can be falsely positive for years after successful completion of treatment (more common in the first 1–2 years), old CXR signs such as cavities and TB scars can make identifying new changes more difficult.
- Compare new imaging with that at the end of the last course of TB treatment.

Acute management

- As for all possible respiratory infections, see ➲ Chapter 23
- Consider early involvement of an infection or respiratory specialist to discuss empirical anti-fungal or TB treatment if index of suspicion is high based on history, severity of presentation, and clinical signs.
- Consider the need for infection control precautions pending microbiology results (respiratory PPE, isolation).

Considerations when reviewing a patient currently receiving tuberculosis treatment

Infection risk

Effective TB treatment rapidly reduces onwards transmission risk. Those with smear-positive TB (i.e. sputum positive for AFB on microscopy), are considered infectious until completion of the first 2 weeks of effective anti-tuberculous chemotherapy.

All other patients with TB are non-infectious unless there are concerns for non-compliance or non-response to treatment. Fig 24.1 shows important clinical considerations when assessing a patient with TB on treatment.

Treatment toxicity

The most frequent side effects of the four most commonly used DS-TB drugs are shown in Table 24.1 and common interactions are shown in Table 24.2. Acute abnormalities in liver or kidney function, significant QTc prolongation, reduction in visual acuity/visual field defects, myositis, could indicate toxicity related to TB drugs.

Depending on the severity of toxicity, doses may need to be reduced or the offending drug(s) stopped.

Look out for:

Worsening clinical condition or CXR changes. Comparison of CXR to previous is recommended.

In some patients, there is an initial worsening of condition (e.g. increased size of lymph nodes or worsening of CXR changes) because of a degree of immune reconstitution (more relevant in HIV/TB co-infection but a milder form can occur if HIV negative). Consider treatment with oral steroids.

Consider concomitant community-or hospital-acquired infection.

Fig. 24.1 Key clinical considerations when assessing a patient undergoing TB. treatment

Drug-induced liver injury

Drug-induced liver injury (DILI) is the most common adverse reaction to anti-TB treatment. The hepatotoxicity is caused by toxic drug metabolites from some anti-TB drugs including rifampicin, isoniazid, and pyrazinamide. Risk factors include age >60 yrs, male gender, HIV, HBV- or HCV-positive status, malnutrition, alcohol intake, concurrent use of potentially hepatotoxic drugs (including herbal remedies).

Liver toxicity is defined as ALT ≥ 5 times the upper limit of normal (5×ULN) or ALT ≥ 3×ULN + total bilirubin > 2×ULN.

Table 24.2 Common interactions with other drugs

Drug	Increases level	Decreases level
Rifampicin*		Oral contraceptive pill Warfarin Phenytoin Carbamazepine Barbiturates Sulphonylureas Corticosteroids Cyclosporin
Isoniazid*	Phenytoin Carbamazepine Warfarin	

*Drug interactions listed in this table are not exhaustive; all concurrent medications should be checked for interactions prior to starting TB treatment.

All would need to be stopped (including ethambutol) and reintroduced one at a time once liver function tests have returned to baseline (starting with ethambutol as lowest associated risk). If the patient is unwell or still smear-positive, second-line therapy should be considered until withheld drugs can be reinstituted.

Advice should be sought from the treating chest or infectious diseases physician and local TB-MDT before any changes to the TB treatment regimen are made.

⓵ Never leave a patient on only one TB-active drug.

Non-tuberculous mycobacteria

Non-tuberculous mycobacteria (NTM) are ubiquitous environmental acid-fast mycobacteria different from mycobacterium tuberculosis complex; found in warm, moist environments (hot-tubs, steam rooms). Over 190 NTM species and sub-species exist, with only a handful known to cause significant pulmonary infection, occurring mostly in people with chronic structural lung disease and immune-compromised states. They are considered non-contagious with no person–person transmission.

They require challenging treatment regimens due to intrinsic resistance to antimicrobials, lack of research defining optimum treatment regimens, and limited interest and funding into new drug development.

Non-tuberculous mycobacteria species causing pulmonary infection

- Mycobacterium avian complex (MAC) made up of *M.avium* and *M.intracellulare* (also known as MAI), most commonly occurring.
- *M.kanasii.*
- *M.abscessus.*
- *M.gordonaii.*
- *M.chelonae.*
- *M.fortuitum.*

Presentation

Often non-specific but frequently report breathlessness, recurrent infections not responding to standard antibiotic regimens, cough, haemoptysis, chest pain, fatigue, weight loss.

Radiologically progressive lung damage on CXR or CT-imaging (consolidation, nodular bronchiectatic changes, cavitation, fibrosis).

Diagnosis

Diagnosis must be confirmed clinically, radiologically, and microbiologically. Thee sets of sputum should be sent for Ziehl-Neelson stain looking for AFB and bacterial culture. If this is negative and infection still suspected then BAL or induced sputum should be performed. Gene sequencing is considered the gold standard.

Modern available rapid molecular methods include: nucleic acid probes, PCR-restricted enzyme analysis (PRA), nucleic acid amplification line probe assay, MALDI-TOF mass spectrometry. High-multiplex molecular genetic assays can differentiate MTB-Complex from NTM and NTM species. There are also histopathological features on lung biopsy samples (necrotising granulomatous inflammation).

① It is important to exclude similarly presenting diagnoses including MTB.

Management

- Early involvement of specialist MDT.
- A confirmed diagnosis does not necessarily warrant immediate treatment initiation.
- Similar to MTB, there is a high propensity of NTM to develop antimicrobial resistance.

- Requires multi-drug regimens (combination oral, inhaled, and intravenous). Drugs used include macrolides (clarithromycin/azithromycin), aminoglycosides (streptomycin, amikacin, tobramycin), carbapenems (imipenem/meropenem), rifampicin/rifabutin, ethambutol.
- Long treatment course (12–24 months or longer in some cases).
- Side effects from treatment are common.

Further reading

1. WHO Global TB Report, 2023.
2. WHO consolidated guidelines on tuberculosis (drug-susceptible and drug-resistant), updated May 2022.
3. British Thoracic Society multi-drug resistance clinical advice service.
4. Treatment of nontuberculous mycobacterial pulmonary disease: an official ATS/ERS/ESCMID/IDSA clinical practice guideline 2020. Available online https://www.idsociety.org/practice-guideline/nontuberculous-mycobacterial-ntm-diseases/
5. BTS Guidelines for the diagnosis and management of NTM 2017.

Chapter 25

Pleural effusion

Introduction

Pleural effusions are a common clinical scenario and can develop because of over 60 different causes including diseases of the pleura or underlying lung, systemic conditions, organ dysfunction, and drugs.

They are defined as an accumulation of fluid between the visceral and parietal pleura. This can result from an increased fluid formation and/or reduced fluid reabsorption. There is normally around 20 ml of fluid present in the pleural space. Around 400 ml needs to be present before clinically apparent, whilst >200 ml is visible on the PA chest radiograph.

Causes

Pleural effusions can be caused by a huge array of different causes, however, large case series have shown that cancer, heart failure, and parapneumonic infections account for most cases.

Divided according to the biochemical characteristics of the fluid into transudate and exudate. Although common transudative causes usually result in bilateral effusions, they may result in a unilateral effusion.

Transudate (protein <30 g/L)

Common

- Left ventricular failure.

Note: acute diuresis can result in borderline exudative features.

- Liver cirrhosis.
- Hypoalbuminaemia (e.g. nephrotic syndrome).

Less common

- Pulmonary embolus.
- Chronic hypothyroidism.
- Malignancy (5% are transudative).
- Constrictive pericarditis.
- Mitral stenosis.
- Nephrotic syndrome.
- Peritoneal dialysis.
- CSF fluid leak into pleural space.

Exudate (protein >30 g/L)

Common

- Parapneumonic effusion/empyema.
- Pulmonary embolus + infarction.
- Malignancy (often secondary or mesothelioma).
- Tuberculosis.
- Trauma (haemothorax).
- Autoimmune pleuritis.

Less common

- Connective tissue disease (rheumatoid, SLE, mixed connective tissues disease, lupus, EGPA, GPA).
- Infectious (hepatitis, cholecystitis, fungal disease, viral pneumonias)
- Inflammatory disorders (pancreatitis, benign asbestos pleural disease, sarcoidosis, ARDS, radiator therapy).
- Iatrogenic/trauma (post-coronary artery bypass graft, oesophageal rupture, haemothorax, enteral feeding tube in pleural space, radiofrequency ablation).
- Drugs (e.g., nitrofurantoin, dantrolene, methysergide, dasatinib, amiodarone, interleukin-2, procarbazine, methotrexate, clozapine, phenytoin, beta blocker).
- Malignancy-related (chylothorax, lymphoma, leukaemia, paraproteinaemia).
- Other (endometriosis, drowning, electrical burns, ovarian hyperstimulation syndrome).

Clinical approach

Thorough history and examination will guide further investigation. A combination of history and examination has been shown to reliably identify transudative causes, obviating the need for immediate diagnostic thoracentesis in some cases.

Symptoms

Ask about:

- Dyspnoea.
  - Common even in small effusions.
  - Due to reduced chest wall compliance and lung compression.
  - Often little shunting/hypoxia.
- Chest pain.
  - Involvement of parietal pleural or chest wall.
  - Often signifies exudative cause.
  - Pleuritic pain in 75% of PE effusions.
- Cough.
  - May be non-specific.
  - Often purulent sputum in empyema.
  - Hemoptysis.
- Fever.
  - Empyema/parapneumonic effusion—recent history of pneumonia.
  - TB—enquire about exposure to TB, travel history, past history of TB.
  - Malignancy (mesothelioma/lymphoma).
- Constitutional.
  - Weight loss, anorexia, malaise, night sweats.
  - Seen in TB/empyema/malignancy.
- Symptoms/risk factors of malignancy.
  - Change in bowel habit, breast lumps, skin abnormalities.
  - Is the patient up-to-date on screening—breast, cervical, bowel cancer.
- Vomiting—risk of ruptured oesophagus.
- Skin/eyes/joints.
  - Consider rheumatological cause.
- Past medical history.
  - Lung conditions that predispose to parapneumonic or malignant effusions (immune deficiency, bronchiectasis, chronic bronchitis).
  - Known cardiac disease.
  - Known liver disease.
  - Known renal disease.
  - Oesophageal disease/intervention.
  - History of trauma/rib fractures.
- Drug history.
  - Large numbers of drugs can cause an effusion: commonly used include tyrosine kinase inhibitors, amiodarone, phenytoin, nitrofurantoin, methotrexate.
  - Consult www.pneumotox.com
- Recent procedures—consider iatrogenic cause.
  - Central line insertion, urinary or biliary intervention, CSF fluid shunt placement, thoracoabdominal surgery.

- Risk factors/occupational history.
  - Exposure to asbestos.
  - Ethnicity and living conditions (TB).
  - Smoking history (malignancy).
  - Risk stratify for embolic disease.

Examination

Features of effusion

- RR and SaO_2 (may be maintained even in moderate effusion).
- Decreased expansion.
- Stony dullness to percussion.
- Decreased breath sounds.
- Decreased vocal resonance and decreased or absent tactile femitus.
- Tracheal/mediastinal shift away if large effusion.
- Large effusion with no mediastinal shift: implies associated lung collapse (bronchial carcinoma) or encasement (mesothelioma).

Features of cause

- Basal crackles, raised JVP, peripheral oedema, S3 (CCF).
- Signs of chronic liver disease.
- Facial and peripheral oedema (nephrotic syndrome).
- Hypoxaemia and tachypnoea despite small effusion (consider PE).
- Pyrexia, unwell, hypotension (empyema or parapneumonic effusion).
- Cachexia, lymphadenopathy (malignancy, empyema, TB).
- Arthropathy, rash, eye disease (rheumatological).
- Signs of recent procedure/surgery (CABG).

Investigations

Bloods

- FBC (anaemia, leukocytosis, elevated WBC in infective process).
- Inflammatory markers (empyema, TB, autoimmune).
- Biochemistry (renal disease, cirrhosis, hypoalbuminaemia).
- Serum total protein, LDH, glucose (paired samples for pleural fluid, see below).
- Clotting (if further intervention is likely, e.g. pleural biopsy, drain insertion).
- Autoantibodies if indicated.
- Serum BNP (if diagnostic doubt about heart failure).
- Blood cultures (if presentation suggests infection).

Chest X-ray

- PA chest X-ray is the first indicated radiological test if effusion is suspected.
- Is the fluid unilateral or bilateral?
- An effusion is normally identified by dependent opacity of the hemithorax with a lateral meniscus.
- Loculated effusions may appear as a rim of lateral shadowing, or as a discrete mass as fluid is encysted within the fissure.
- In the setting of a supine patient (e.g. ICU + ventilated) effusion may appear as a hazy opacification of a hemithorax or thickening of the fissure.

- Look for clues to aetiology (rib fractures, consolidation, lymphadenopathy, discrete mass).
- An effusion as small as 50 ml can be seen on a lateral film and around 200 ml will be visible on PA film.

Thoracic ultrasound (TUS)

- TUS should be performed on every patient at their initial presentation and again whenever a pleural procedure is being performed.
- TUS immediately prior to intervention is strongly advocated. It improves diagnostic accuracy and improves the safety of invasive procedures.
- The initial TUS evaluation should confirm presence of pleural fluid and can help with guiding on size and character of the effusion.
- USS signs of malignancy with nodularity seen on the diaphragm and parietal pleural is highly suggestive of malignant pleural effusion.

Thoracic CT scan

- If the above tests on pleural fluid are non-diagnostic (e.g. exudate of unknown cause), thoracic CT is the investigation of choice.
- Performed before drainage of effusion and with IV contrast to enable visualisation of pleural abnormalities.
- CT is valuable in the diagnosis of malignant and infective pleural disease, and reliably differentiates lung abscess from empyema.
- CT features which are more common in pleural infection over malignancy are: lentiform configuration of pleural fluid, visceral pleural thickening, hypertrophy of extrapleural fat, increased density of the extrapleural fat, and presence of pulmonary consolidation.
- Of note, in around 5% of cases malignancy can coexist with pleural infection. CT follow up (for up to 2 years) should be considered for patients with pleural infection to exclude occult malignancy if there is clinical concern.

Positron emission tomography-CT (PET CT)

- The role of PET CT in predicting malignancy in patients with pleural effusion or pleural thickening is still debated. It may be helpful in selected patients.
- A suspicious PET CT may support identification of optimal biopsy site and identify primary tumour.

Thoracic MRI scan

- MRI can provide better imaging of soft tissue. This can be helpful if there is concern about tumour invasion into chest wall or diaphragm.

Pleural fluid investigations

When to conduct a diagnostic thoracocentesis?

Pleural fluid analysis is the key to making a precise diagnosis and guides further investigation and management. All pleural effusions of unknown cause should be sampled, except where a transudative cause is diagnosed clinically (e.g. bilateral effusions in clinical context of left ventricular failure).

Current guidelines recommend using real-time USS guidance for all pleural procedures. A 50 ml syringe with a 21G needle under sterile conditions would be used to obtain a diagnostic sample (➔ Chapter 51). 20–50 ml of pleural fluid should be submitted for cytological assessment and it is recommended that pleural fluid should be sent in both plain and blood culture bottle tubes in patients with suspected pleural infections.

If the effusion is small or has atypical features on the CXR (e.g. loculations), radiological guidance may be needed with support from interventional radiology.

Pleural fluid appearance

- Commonly clear and straw-coloured in transudates and some exudates.
- Frank pus.
  - Diagnoses empyema.
  - Immediate action required (intercostal drainage, antibiotics).
- Turbid.
  - Consider empyema or chylothorax.
- Bloodstained.
  - Malignancy/infarction/trauma.
  - True haemothorax will quickly clot in the sampling tube.
  - If in doubt, pleural fluid haematocrit >50% serum haematocrit is diagnostic of haemothorax.
- Food particles.
  - Diagnostic of oesophageal rupture.
  - Immediate action required.

Biochemistry

Immediately send fluid for:

- Protein.
- LDH.
- Glucose.
- pH (via blood gas analyser)—unless fluid is excessively turbid and likely to break the blood gas analyser!

Transudate versus exudate

A protein level <25 g/L is a definite transudate and >35 g/L a definite exudate. Between 25 and 35 g/L, or if the serum protein level is abnormal, further assessment is required using Light's criteria:

- pleural fluid protein to serum ratio >0.5.
- pleural fluid LDH to serum ratio >0.6.
- pleural fluid LDH > two-thirds upper limit of normal serum range.

One or more of these criteria is reliably diagnostic of an exudative effusion.

Pleural fluid pH

- Used in the diagnosis of complicated parapneumonic effusion requiring drainage (<7.2).
- Local anaesthetics are acidic and will change the measured value.
- Low pH also seen in malignancy, TB, oesophageal rupture, connective tissue diseases including RA.
- Analysis should be by blood gas machine.

Pleural fluid glucose

- Mirrors pleural fluid pH and can be used if pH not available.
- Normally follows serum glucose.
- Low (<3.3 mmol/L) in empyema, TB, rheumatoid effusion, and malignancy.
- Difficult to interpret in patient with hyperglycaemia.

Microbiology

The presence of bacteria in the pleural space is always abnormal and diagnostic of pleural infection, even in the absence of biochemical criteria. A sample should be sent for:

- Gram stain.
- Culture + sensitivity.
- If TB is suspected send for: acid-alcohol fast bacilli and TB culture (takes up to 9 weeks and yield from pleural fluid is not very high).

Sending pleural fluid in aerobic and anaerobic blood culture bottled in addition to standard culture can increase microbial yield.

Cell count + cytology

Cell count

May aid in narrowing the differential diagnosis:

- Neutrophil predominant (>50%): suggests an acute process.
- Eosinophilic (>10%): non-specific, may imply air or blood in the pleural space.
- Lymphocyte predominant (>50%): may suggest TB or malignancy. Most chronic effusions will be predominantly lymphocytic. Lymphocyte population of >90% is likely lymphoma or TB.

Cytology

- Diagnostic of malignancy in 60% of cases.
- Yield may be increased by a second diagnostic tap.

Special tests

- Pleural fluid amylase should be requested in suspected oesophageal rupture or pancreatitis. Isoenzyme analysis will confirm oesophageal rupture (amylase of salivary origin).
- Pleural fluid adenosine deaminase (ADA) level and interferon gamma (IFN-gamma) can be sent if TB effusion is suspected, ADA level of >40 U/L is highly suggestive.

- Pleural fluid cholesterol and triglycerides should be sent in suspected chylothorax (interruption of the thoracic duct leading to chyle leak into the pleural space). Raised triglycerides and normal cholesterol suggest chylothorax, raised cholesterol and normal triglycerides suggest pseudo-chylothorax (generally a complication or evolution of chronic exudative effusions).
- Pleural fluid NT-proBNP can be helpful in diagnosing heart failure in patients with a unilateral pleural effusion. Serum NT-proBNP can also be helpful.
- Pleural fluid ANA can support diagnosis of lupus pleural effusion.

Further tests

- Thoracoscopy can be used for diagnostic purposes in those in which there is diagnostic uncertainty. Medical thoracoscopy can be carried out by respiratory physicians or referral to local thoracic surgeons.
- Pleural biopsy (image-guided, or thoracoscopic) may be required: specialist referral is recommended.
- Bronchoscopy has no role in the investigation of pleural effusion, unless an endobronchial lesion associated with collapse is suspected.
- Tumour marker testing in pleural fluid is an emerging field. Positive results for markers such as CA 15-3, CA 19-9, mesothelin, and CYFRA21-1 may demonstrate the presence of a neoplastic process.

Management

Transudates

- Successful management of the underlying disease process will usually result in resolution of the pleural effusion, without recourse to intercostal drainage or further interventions.
- Therapeutic thoracocentesis may be required for short-term symptomatic relief. Removal of as little as 300 ml of fluid (even from a large effusion) may decompress the effusion and ameliorate symptoms.

Exudates

Management depends on cause.

- Traumatic haemothorax: guidelines suggest insertion of a large bore (>18F) chest drain and the space drained to dryness.
- Pleural infection: requires prompt chest drain insertion and antibiotic therapy.
- Oesophageal rupture: associated with a risk of mediastinitis and pleural infection. Patient should be nil by mouth, and a surgical/ gastroenterological opinion sought.
- The undiagnosed effusion: if, despite investigation, the cause of effusion remains obscure, TB and PE should be considered (specific therapy available).

Chapter 26

Pleural infection

Introduction

Pleural infection (empyema and complicated parapneumonic effusion) remains a common medial problem with a yearly incidence of 11.2 cases per 100 000 population. It continues to cause a considerable burden to the NHS.

A pleural effusion occurs in up to 40% of cases of pneumonia. The majority of these will resolve with treatment of the pneumonia, but a subset will undergo bacterial invasion and subsequent infection will be established.

Pleural infections are seen in approximately 2–3% of all pneumonias; rates are highest in hospitalised patients and there is a suggestion from recent epidemiological studies that rates may be slowly rising. Common risk factors for pleural infections include partially treated pneumonia, influenza, immunosuppression, age <18 years and >65, aspiration, poor dental hygiene, and drug/alcohol abuse.

Despite improved understanding of the aetiology, pathophysiology, and advances in management of pleural infections, clinical outcomes remain poor. Up to 20% of patients die within 12 months of a pleural infection and approximately 15% of cases require invasive thoracic surgery.

Early recognition and prompt treatment is important to prevent progression to disease only amenable to surgical treatment.

Some cases of pleural infection are not associated with an underlying pneumonia, most notably iatrogenic and traumatic aetiologies.

Definitions

Pleural infection

Pleural infection is defined as bacterial entry and replication in the pleural space.

Parapneumonic effusion

Parapneumonic effusion (PPE) refers to the accumulation of fluid in the pleural space in the context of adjacent pneumonia.

- An uncomplicated or simple PPE refers to an effusion with no biochemical or microbiological evidence of bacterial invasion, which is free flowing.
- A complicated PPE effusion refers to an effusion with biochemical evidence of bacterial invasion.

Empyema

Empyema refers to the collection of frank pus (macroscopic detection of purulent fluid) within the pleural space. This can develop when bacteria, fungi, parasites, or mycobacteria invade the pleural space.

Pleural infection

Effusion with microbiological evidence of bacterial invasion (even if no biochemical parameters consistent with bacterial invasion).

Complex effusion

Complex effusion refers to those with internal loculations.

Uniloculated effusion

Uniloculated effusion refers to an effusion which is free flowing or fixed and without loculations.

Pathophysiology

Pleural infection develops because of host response to inflammation and bacterial invasion. It is thought that pleural infection develops in three stages:

- Stage 1 (exudative stage): Bacterial infection of the lung is established with associated inflammation and cytokine production. Inflammation at the visceral pleural surface results in increased capillary permeability. Interstitial fluid increases due to the pneumonia and moves across into the visceral pleural space. A simple or uncomplicated PPE would be seen at this stage.
- Stage 2 (complicated PPE and empyema): Bacteria invasion occurs across the damaged pleural mesothelium, resulting in biochemical changes without formation of frank pus (complicated PPE). When infection is established, it can lead to the production of frank pus (empyema, a combination of dead organisms and leukocytes).
- Bacteria in the pleural space stimulates an inflammatory response resulting in fibrin deposition; due to this septations and loculations form. Of note the fluid characteristics may be different between loculations.
- Stage 3 (chronic organisation): If infection persists, fibrosis occurs with the formation of a chronically infected thick 'peel' over the visceral and parietal pleura. This can stop full re-expansion of the lung leading to trapped lung and impaired lung function. This thickened pleura often resolves over time but in some cases can be permanent.

Some cases of pleural infection are not associated with an underlying pneumonia, this results from a pathogen directly inoculating or invading the pleural space. The most likely causes of these include oesophageal rupture, chest trauma, hematogenous spread, post-surgical complications (e.g. bronchopleural fistula), or extension from sources outside the thorax such as liver abscess.

There is a wide spectrum of potential pathogens that cause pleural infections; these vary depending on the underlying cause of the pleural infection. The common bacterial causes of community-acquired pneumonia are commonly causative pathogens in pleural infection, namely *Streptococcus pneumoniae* and *Staphylococcus aureus*. Pleural infections arising from aspiration are often polymicrobial with a mix of oral *streptococci* and anaerobes. Fungal pleural infections are rare, *Candida* species are responsible for the majority of cases, less commonly *Aspergillus* species and *cryptococcus* can be seen.

Acute presentation

History

- Pleuritic pain is common but not universal.
- Cough +/- sputum production and dyspnoea are common symptoms.
- Sweats and fevers.
- Weight loss, anorexia, and malaise.
- Symptoms may be present for a few days or several months.
- History of previous transthoracic procedures, chest trauma, or upper GI surgery/interventional endoscopy.

Risk factors

- Diabetes mellitus.
- Alcohol abuse.
- Intravenous drug use.
- Gastro-oesophageal reflux disease.
- Aspiration risk.

Examination

- Fever (not universal).
- Tachypnoea, sweaty.
- Cachexia if long history.
- Signs of pleural effusion may be present; dullness on percussion, decreased breath sounds, and decreased fremitus (may be difficult to detect clinically if loculated collection).

Other presentations

- Pneumonia not resolving on treatment: request repeat/further radiology to assess for the presence of pleural fluid. Especially in patients with risk factors for empyema (e.g. aspiration), persistent or new fevers, and poor response despite adequate antibiotic coverage.
- Patients with weight loss, anorexia, fevers, and an abnormal CXR (often mistaken for malignancy): more commonly caused by anaerobic organisms.
- After oesophageal instrumentation/surgery, spontaneous oesophageal perforation (Boerhaeve's syndrome).
- After previous chest drain insertion/pleural procedure (e.g. pneumothorax, drainage of malignant effusion).

Investigations

Laboratory investigations

- Raised white cell count, CRP, ESR.
- Anaemia of chronic disease if long history.
- Other potential helpful tests include sputum culture, urine for *S.pneumoniae* antigen testing, interferon-gamma release assays for TB, galactomannan, and cryptococcal antigen.

Chest radiograph

- May reveal typical features of a small, moderate, or large effusion.
- The presence of pleural fluid in a non-dependent area on the CXR (e.g. lateral collection) makes empyema more likely.
- May present as enlarging mass (encysted fluid in fissure).
- Loculated posterior collections may not be readily identified as pleural fluid.
- Raised hemidiaphragm may be associated with underlying lung collapse and is difficult to appreciate with effusion present.

Thoracic ultrasound

- Once pleural fluid has been detected on chest radiography, thoracic ultrasound should be used to evaluate the nature of the effusion and for assessment of possibility of sampling or drain insertion.
- Thoracic ultrasound is typically preformed at the bedside to allow for real time ultrasound prior to any pleural procedures.

CT chest

Request if atypical features as above on the chest radiograph and/or thoracic ultrasound. Typically preformed with IV contrast to help identify the pleural membranes.

- Defines 3D anatomy of the pleural space.
- Can easily appreciate loculations, pleural and parenchymal abnormalities, and other causes of pleural infections such as oesophageal rupture and bronchopleural fistula.
- Permits image-guided catheter insertion.
- Reliably differentiates pulmonary abscess from pleural infection.

Pleural fluid sampling + analysis

When to sample pleural fluid?

- All patients with an effusion in the context of pneumonia, a febrile illness, or recent chest trauma/instrumentation require pleural fluid sampling. This is the key diagnostic step, and the results alter immediate management.

Key points

- The use of ultrasound guidance immediately prior to thoracentesis is required in all cases; it reduces the risk of complications and improves the rate of successful fluid sampling.
- There is no definition of what is considered a 'safe' amount for sampling, the decision often lies with the ultrasonographer. Most experts would usually consider a pleural space of >1 cm safe.

- It is preferred that the same needle/syringe used to anaesthetise should not collect the pH sample; residual lidocaine and heparin can falsely decrease the pH and air in the syringe can falsely increase the pH.
- In patients with suspected pleural infection, pleural fluid should be sent to microbiology in both plain (white top) container and volumes of 5–10 ml inoculated into blood culture bottles (anaerobic and aerobic).
- In cases where smaller volumes of fluid are obtained, 2–5 ml should be prioritised to blood culture bottles rather than plain, sterile containers.

Assess pleural fluid for

- Appearance (frank pus/turbid fluid = empyema).
- Pleural fluid pH via blood gas analyser—within 1 hour of sampling.
- Gram stain, culture, and sensitivity.
- Protein/glucose/LDH.
- Cytology including cell count.

Pleural fluid pH

This investigation differentiates simple from complicated PPE and therefore guides which pleural collections require drainage. pH should not be requested on frankly purulent fluid (may damage blood gas analysers and the result will not alter management).

Studies suggest that those PPEs with a lower pH (<7.2) run a more 'complicated' course, requiring chest drainage ± surgical intervention for resolution.

- Pleural fluid pH <7.2 diagnoses complicated PPE; indicates the need for prompt chest tube drainage.
- Not every effusion with a low pH is a complicated PPE (other causes include malignancy, TB, rheumatoid); the context must be considered.
- Not every pleural effusion with a pH >7.2 will run a 'simple' course. Regular review is required and if there is lack of clinical improvement or worsening, a repeat pH sample is advised.
- It is sometimes necessary to institute chest tube drainage in a normal pH effusion (i.e. simple PPE) if this is causing respiratory embarrassment.
- If pH is not available, low pleural fluid glucose (<3.3 mmol/L) may be used as an indicator of high likelihood of complicated PPE/ pleural infection and can be used to inform decision making to insert chest drain.
- Alternative diagnoses that can mimic PPE with low pH and potential loculations need to be considered such as rheumatoid effusions, effusions due to advanced malignancy/mesothelioma.

Pleural fluid biochemistry

PPE begins as an exudate (as defined before) but during the simple PPE stage the biochemical characteristics are normal. As bacterial invasion occurs, biochemical changes occur to produce:

- low glucose (<2.2 mmol/L)
- high LDH (>1000 IU/L)
- low pH (<7.2)

These changes are seen because of a combination of high metabolic activity, rapid cell turnover, and lactate production.

Pleural fluid microbiology

Essential to send a sample for microbiology as soon as possible, preferably prior to starting antibiotics but thoracentesis should not delay prompt antimicrobial therapy.

- Combined Gram stain and culture is only positive in around 60% of cases; hence empirical antibiotics required.
- Blood cultures are positive in 12% of cases and should be conducted in all suspected cases (may be the only positive culture).

The microbiology of pleural infection is varied and there are substantial differences between hospital and community-acquired disease. The organisms represent a wider range of pathogens than that seen in pneumonia, with several organisms resistant to 'standard' antibiotics for pneumonia.

Most common community-acquired organisms

- *Streptococcus milleri.*
- *Streptococcus pneumoniae.*
- Anaerobes.
- *Staphylococci.*

Most common hospital-acquired organisms

- MRSA (up to one-third of cases).
- *Staphylococci.*
- Gram-negative bacteria (e.g. *Enterobacter*).
- *Pseudomonas.*
- Anaerobes.

Cytology

Malignancy can cause pleural fluid acidosis, therefore sending fluid for assessment of malignancy cells is important. In addition, cytological examination for appropriate stains can be sent for diagnosis of some specific organisms such as mycobacteria, *actinomyces*, and *nocardia*.

Management

Risk stratification

- Understanding which patients are at higher risk of poor outcomes following pleural infection may support clinicians' decision making.
- Greater risk of adverse outcomes are seen in healthcare-acquired pleural infections and the presence of complex effusions.
- RAPID risk stratification scoring system is advised by BTS to aid in patient discussions about potential outcomes. It considers serum urea, pleural fluid purulence, infection source, age of the patient, and serum albumin levels and risk stratified into low-, medium-, and high-risk patients.

Antibiotic therapy

- All patients with suspected pleural infection should receive broad-spectrum antibiotics.
- Empirical therapy is required initially until culture results are available. In 40% , no organism is found; thus, empirical antibiotics are required for the entire treatment course. Antibiotic selection varies based on the site of acquisition, i.e. community- versus hospital-acquired, severity, local epidemiology, and patient's past bacterial profile.
- Do not delay initiating antibiotics whilst waiting for culture results. Start as soon as diagnosis established clinically, and cultures taken. Antibiotics should not be deferred pending thoracentesis if there is likely to be a delay in performing this procedure.
- Antibiotics should be rationalised in the light of positive culture results.
- The optimal length of antibiotic therapy is not known. This is often decided on a patient-by-patient basis depending on type of effusion, adequacy of drainage, response to treatment, and patient risk factors. Most authorities treat for 2–3 weeks for complicated PPE and between 4–6 weeks for empyema (with IV therapy initially which can be switched to oral regime when clinical response is clear and no further drainage procedures are needed).

Empirical antibiotic regimens

Antibiotic choices will be governed by local microbiology and local practice. Suggested empirical regimens are given below, providing broad-spectrum cover for possible organisms.

Community-acquired infection

- Second-generation cephalosporin (e.g. cefuroxime) + anaerobic cover (e.g. metronidazole).
- If penicillin allergic, meropenem 1 g tds IV + metronidazole (po 400 mg tds or IV 500 mg tds).
- Oral treatment: amoxicillin + clavulanic acid (co-amoxiclav).
- In cases of suspected *Legionella*, a macrolide should be added.

Hospital-acquired infection

- Cover required for MRSA, Gram-negative organisms, and anaerobes, e.g. piperacillin-tazobactam 4.5g TDS or meropenem 1 g tds IV + vancomycin 1 g bd IV.
- Oral treatment is not appropriate.

Chest tube drainage

Intercostal drainage is required for:

- Empyema (pus/turbid fluid).
- Microbiologically proven infection (pleural Gram stain or culture positive).
- Complicated PPE (pH < 7.2).
- Large free-flowing effusions, i.e. >0.5 hemithorax.
- Effusions associated with thickened parietal pleura.
- Sepsis from pleural source.

Chest drain should be considered in patients with pH >7.2 and <7.4 (intermediate risk of pleural infection or complicated PPE), if LDH >900 IU/L and other clinical parameters suggest complicated PPE.

Chest drain size

- Small (10–14F) and large (24F+) chest drains may be used.
- Chest tube bore size appears to have no effect on outcomes but bore size >14F is likely to increase post-treatment pain. Due to this it is recommended that initial drainage should be undertaken by a small-bore chest tube.
- If smaller drains are used, regular flushes (e.g. sterile saline 20 ml qds) are recommended.
- Chest drains can generally be removed when drainage volumes fall below 50–100 ml/day for 2–3 days, imaging shows good response, and the patient is clinically improving.

Radiologically guided drains

- Image-guided drain insertion is often required given the complexities of pleural space anatomy, loculated/septated fluid, and encysted collections seen in pleural infection.
- A low threshold for referral for image-guided drainage is recommended in cases of failed drain insertion at the bedside.

Intrapleural therapy

Intrapleural treatments have been used for many years in an attempt to reduce septations and hence improve drainage.

Combination tissue plasminogen activator (TPA) and DNAse appears to reduce hospital length of stay and should be considered for the treatment of pleural infection in patients with persistent pleural collection despite chest tube drainage.

Saline irrigation can also be considered for those unsuitable for surgical intervention or intrapleural fibrinolytics.

Drain management

- If drainage stops in the absence of CXR resolution or improved clinical state of the patient, further imaging is recommended to assess drain position.
- Drain repositioning/reinsertion may be required.

Further management

- Patients with pleural infection should be under the care of a respiratory physician.

- Further management options are surgical and require specialist referral, e.g. video-assisted thoracic surgery (VATS) debridement is indicated in symptomatic patients with a pleural infection that fails to resolve with antibiotic therapy and drainage.

Pneumothorax

Definitions

Pneumothorax is defined as air in the pleural space. It may occur as a result of trauma, causative medical intervention, or spontaneously. Spontaneous pneumothorax can be further divided into primary and secondary.

Spontaneous pneumothorax (SP) is an increasing problem, with annual hospital admissions rising to 14.1 from 9.1 per 100 000 population over the last 50 years.

Any pneumothorax may result in a tension pneumothorax, which requires immediate intervention to prevent rapid deterioration and potentially death. There remains significant mortality from all causes of pneumothorax.

Primary spontaneous pneumothorax

Primary spontaneous pneumothorax (PSP) has an average annual incidence of 19 in 100 000 in males and 8.1 in 100 000 females. Most common in men aged 15–34 years.

Pathophysiology

Although PSP occurs in otherwise healthy lungs, CT imaging often demonstrates emphysema-like pulmonary changes. These small areas of abnormally dilated air spaces (subpleural blebs and bullae) are commonly found in apical areas of lung where pneumothorax has occurred. These areas are thought to rupture, leading to air escaping from the lung into the pleural space.

Risk factors

- Smoking is the most important risk factor with men who smoke increasing their pneumothorax risk by 22-fold and female smokers 9-fold compared with non-smokers.
- Tall and thin body habitus: greater pressure at apical blebs.
- There may also be a familial component in addition to well-known associations including Marfan syndrome, Ehlers-Danlos syndrome, and homocystinuria.

Prognosis

- Risk of recurrence after first episode of PSP is reported to be between 10–30% between 1 and 5 years, with highest risk occurring in the first year.
- Female sex is associated with increased recurrence.
- Smoking cessation with a four-fold decrease in risk of recurrence. Continued smoking increases the risk of recurrence (directly related to amount smoked), up to 100× in some studies of heavy smokers.
- Following first recurrence, without intervention, a third and fourth pneumothorax event can be expected in around 60% and 80% of patients, respectively. Patients are also at higher risk of a contralateral PSP.
- PSP has a very low mortality in the absence of tension pneumothorax (in contrast with secondary pneumothorax).

Secondary spontaneous pneumothorax

Patients can be characterised with secondary spontaneous pneumothorax (SSP) if they are older than 50 years of age and have a smoking history, in addition to the below associated respiratory conditions.

Cystic lung disease

- Emphysema/COPD—most common.
- Asthma.
- Cystic fibrosis.
- *Pneumocystis jiroveci* pneumonia (PJP).
- Interstitial lung disease including IPF, Langerhans cell histiocytosis (LCH), and lymphangiomyomatosis (LAM).

Parenchymal necrosis

- Lung abscess, necrotic pneumonia, TB, fungal disease, septic emboli.
- Cavitating neoplasm.
- Radiation necrosis.
- Pulmonary infarction.

Other

- Catamenial pneumothorax; recurrent SP during menstruation, associated with endometriosis of pleura.
- Pleuroparenchymal fibroelastosis.

Prognosis

- Risk of recurrence after first episode of SSP is around 13–39% .
- Large air leaks more common with associated complications.
- Mortality 10% : therefore, aggressive management.

Acute presentation

Initial questions

- Any evidence of tension pneumothorax (see below)? If so, manage immediately.
- Is the patient truly breathless (not just shallow breathing due to pleuritic pain)?
- Is there evidence of underlying lung disease?

History

- Chest pain: sudden onset, often pleuritic and usually preceding other symptoms (thought to be secondary to ripping of adhesions between visceral and parietal pleura).
- Breathlessness: sudden onset. May not be present in patients with small pneumothorax (especially primary) but may be severe and present as an acute on chronic exacerbation (e.g. COPD).
- Duration of symptoms: almost 50% of patients have symptoms of pneumothorax for 2 days before presenting. A long history should not put you off the diagnosis and may be associated with re-expansion pulmonary oedema.
- Previous history of lung disease and chronic respiratory symptoms.
- Previous episodes and previous treatments.
- Previous history of trauma (may present sometime after traumatic event): consider traumatic pneumothorax. Occurs secondary to penetrating chest trauma (includes rib fracture), deceleration injury of the lung and/or increased intrathoracic pressure (e.g. blunt chest trauma) leading to alveolar rupture.
- Consider iatrogenic pneumothorax after the following:
    - Chest aspiration.
    - Subclavian central line insertion.
    - Transbronchial biopsy at bronchoscopy.
    - Image-guided lung biopsy.
    - Positive pressure ventilation (may occur in the absence of chest instrumentation/trauma).
    - Pacemaker insertion.
    - Intercostal nerve block.
    - Chest compression (NB post-resuscitation).

Examination

- If tracheal deviation away from the affected side and shocked patient (low blood pressure, tachycardia, cardiovascular collapse), tension pneumothorax has occurred and requires immediate action (see next section).
- For patients with smaller SP (less than 15% of the hemithorax) the examination may be unremarkable.
- For larger SP (>15%) there may be decreased or absent breath sounds, reduced chest wall movement, and hyper-resonance of the affected side.
- Tachycardia is one of the most common physical examination findings but is non-specific. Jugular venous distention and pulsus paradoxus can also be seen.

Tension pneumothorax

This is a medical emergency: do not request further investigations (e.g. CXR).

- Occurs due to a one-way valve in the visceral pleura allowing air from the lung into the pleural space with each inspiration, progressively increasing pleural pressure.
- Increased pleural pressure causes mediastinal shift and diaphragm inversion, eventually resulting in compromised right ventricular filling, cardiovascular collapse, and EMD arrest.
- May occur in pneumothoraces of any size.

Risk factors for tension pneumothorax include:

- Ventilated patients including use of non-invasive ventilation.
- Trauma patients, specifically patients with penetrating chest wounds or post-CPR.
- Patients with chest drains—blocked drain can cause tension pneumothorax to develop.

The patient

- Agitation, respiratory distress, hypoxia.
- Severe chest pain, sweating.
- Hypotension, tachycardia, weak pulse.
- Raised JVP, tracheal deviation (away from side with pneumothorax).
- Decreased expansion, reduced or absent breath sounds, and hyper-resonant on affected side.
- Loss of consciousness.
- PEA arrest.

Immediate management

- Cardiac arrest/emergency team call.
- High-flow oxygen.
- Decompress the hemithorax.
  - Insert large bore cannula (at least 4.5 cm long) into second intercostal space in mid-clavicular line on the side of signs.
  - Hiss of air on entering the pleural space confirms diagnosis.
  - Aspirate until patient stable (relief may occur only a few seconds after initial hiss).
  - Note: almost two-thirds of patients have chest walls thicker than 3 cm. Therefore a cannula at least 4.5 cm long is recommended.
- Definitive management: leave cannula in place as definitive intercostal drain is placed (should not be placed anteriorly; place in mid-axillary line).

Investigations

Chest X-ray

A standard PA chest X-ray should be booked first; in cases where pneumothorax is suspected but not seen on the standard frontal chest radiograph, further X-rays can be considered:

- Lateral decubitus radiography; done with suspected side up, lung should then 'fall' away from chest wall.
- Expiratory chest radiography: lung becomes smaller and denser and therefore pneumothorax can potentially become easier to identify.

Diagnostic in most cases, look for:

- A visible rim between lung margin and chest wall
- Absence of lung markings peripherally between lung margin and chest wall.
- Look for signs of surgical emphysema in skin.
- Blunting of costophrenic angle on side of pneumothorax (small effusion due to bleed).
- Evidence of developing tension (deviated trachea, mediastinal shift, depressed hemidiaphragm).
- Evidence of underlying lung disease.

Size classification

Current guidelines no longer advise management decisions according to size of pneumothorax.

There are various well validated descriptive methods for estimating the percentage volume of pneumothorax from an erect PA CXR including.

The Collins method is commonly used: % = 4.2 + 4.7 (A + B + C)

- A is the maximum apical interpleural distance.
- B is the interpleural distance at midpoint of upper half of lung.
- C is the interpleural distance at midpoint of lower half of lung.

Other validated methods are the Rhea method and Light index.

Pitfalls

- Substantial subcutaneous emphysema.
- Differentiating between a large bulla and a pneumothorax.
- On supine CXR, pneumothoraces may only manifest as increased lucency of the chest ± sharply delineated heart border. Also look for the deep sulus sign, the costophrenic angle is abnormally deepened when the pleural air collects laterally.
- Very small pneumothoraces are reliably detected by a lateral decubitus CXR.

Ultrasound

Chest ultrasound can be used to support diagnosis especially in patients in which X-ray or CT imaging cannot be obtained. It requires specialist expertise. Signs of pneumothorax include:

- Barcode sign (in M mode) where there is a pattern of parallel horizontal lines above and below the pleural line.
- Absence of sliding lung sign.
- Presence of a 'lung point' (point where two pleural layers rejoin from a pneumothorax) and 'A line' sign (horizontal lines below the pleura due to presence of air).

CT chest

Considered the gold standard for diagnosis but is rarely needed and only ordered in cases of diagnostic uncertainty, for example where subcutaneous emphysema obscures the chest radiograph and for the differentiation of bullae and pneumothoraces. Often used in cases of high-impact trauma to detect unsuspected pneumothorax.

Blood tests

Full blood count and clotting screen are helpful to send off urgently because correction of significant anaemia and correction of any clotting abnormalities (INR ≥1.5 or platelets ≤50 x 10^9/L) should be done before inserting a chest drain in patients who are not critically unwell.

ABGs

Not a required investigation in every case. Majority will show evidence of hypoxia, and many will have respiratory alkalosis due to hyperventilation. Some patients with underlying lung disease may have an element of hypercapnia but respiratory acidosis due to this would warrant escalation urgently to senior colleague.

Management

Management is based on:

- The presence of clinical symptoms.
- The presence of any high-risk features (haemodynamic compromise, significant hypoxia, bilateral pneumothorax, underlying lung disease, over 50 years of age with smoking history and haemopneumothorax).
- Patient preference.

Conservative care

Conservative management can be considered in patients with PSP for the treatment of asymptomatic or minimally symptomatic patients regardless of size of pneumothorax.

In patients who are asymptomatic with a SSP, conservative management can also be considered. Patients with PSP can be discharged with initial outpatient review (every 2–4 days); for patients with SSP initial monitoring should be carried out as an inpatient. Once the pneumothorax is considered stable then a 2–4-week OPD follow up can be arranged.

Observation is not recommended for any patient with high-risk features regardless of the size of pneumothorax. These patients will need intervention.

Interventions

When deciding whether to intervene, it is important to consider the individual risks of intervention. Whether it is of sufficient size to intervene depends on clinical context but, in general ≥2 cm laterally or apically on a plain CXR is considered safe. If a CT has been carried out, and with radiological support, a smaller pneumothorax could potentially undergo pleural intervention.

Ambulatory device

Ambulatory treatment using a purpose-made device containing a one-way valve, or Heimlich valve attached to chest drain has the potential to allow outpatient management of pneumothorax.

Ambulatory management should be considered for the treatment of PSP in adults with good support in centres with available expertise and follow-up facilities. Patients need to be followed up initially every 2–4 days until pneumothorax resolution and devise removal, then OPD follow up 2–4 weeks following resolution. There appears to be reduction in length of hospital stay with ambulatory devices but this does not affect rates of recurrence, rates of re-admission, need for further pleural procedures, or complication rates.

Needle aspiration

➲ Chapter 48 for practical procedure.

- For patients with PSP who are mildly symptomatic but with no high-risk features, needle aspiration (NA) can be considered as an alternative to intercostal drainage insertion (ICD).
- Evidence suggests that there is no difference in rates of recurrence or overall complication rates between NA and ICD, however, there appears to be greater need for further plural procedures following NA in patients with PSP.

- The BTS pleural guidance gives both NA and ICD as options for patients whose preference is rapid symptom relief where an ambulatory pathway is not appropriate.
- Aspiration should be stopped if substantial pain or cough occurs or if >2.5 L of air is aspirated (implies ongoing air leak).
- Newer treatments: catheter aspiration of simple pneumothorax (CASP) involves passing an 8F catheter which can be repeatedly aspirated and easily removed. Ambulatory treatment is sometimes used with Heimlich or flutter valves.

Intercostal drainage

➲ Chapter 49 for practical procedure.

- The majority of PSPs do not require intercostal drainage.
- Drainage is associated with a significant rate of morbidity (incorrect placement, infection, bleeding).
- First-line treatment for patients with any high-risk features (detailed above), after failed aspiration or when patient is symptomatic and prefers rapid relief of symptoms using ICD.
- Smaller (10–14F) tubes are usually adequate; larger (>24F) tubes may be required (air leak or subcutaneous emphysema).
- Never clamp a bubbling chest drain (conversion to tension).
- Chemical pleurodesis can be considered for the prevention of recurrent SSP; this can be used during or after first event in patients who are likely to significantly decompensate in the presence of a pneumothorax.

Thoracic surgery

- Thoracic surgery should be considered for patients after the second ipsilateral episode of SP or first contralateral SP to reduce subsequent further recurrences. Surgery can be considered at initial presentation if recurrence prevention is deemed important (e.g. patients presenting with tension pneumothorax, or those in high-risk occupations).

In patients with persistent/prolonged air leak and/or failure of the lung to re-expand on CXR, referral to thoracic surgeons for definitive treatment should be considered. In patients not fit for surgery there is limited evidence available; treatment options to consider include application of suction, conversion to larger-bore chest drain, blood patch or chemical pleurodesis and endobronchial valves.

Post-treatment advice

- Written and verbal advice should be given to patients that they should return to AED if they develop further breathlessness following conservative or active management for SP.
- Patients with an ongoing pneumothorax must not fly. After radiologically proven resolution, they may fly after 7 days.
- After any pneumothorax, the patient may NEVER dive (using compressed air) unless a definitive surgical treatment is conducted.
- Smoking influences the risk of recurrence so cessation should be advised and follow up with a respiratory physician should be arranged for all patients.

Special considerations

Pregnancy

- If asymptomatic and pneumothorax <2 cm in size conservative management can be used, otherwise NA or ICD is recommended.
- Oxygen consumption can increase by 50% during labour and Valsalva manoeuvres during spontaneous delivery can increase size of pneumothorax.
- Both spontaneous delivery and C-section have been associated with increased risk of recurrence, elective assisted delivery with regional anaesthesia may be the safest method of delivery.

Catamenial pneumothorax

- Typically, chest pain, dyspnoea, and haemoptysis within 72 hours before or after menstruation.
- Patients often have a history of endometriosis and pneumothorax is often right sided.
- Management options include hormonal treatment or surgery.

Pneumothorax in cystic fibrosis

- SSP is a common complication of CF occurring in 0.64% of patients per year; patients have higher risk of recurrence.
- Partial pleurectomy is generally regarded as treatment of choice for patient recurrent SSP or chemical pleurodesis in patients not fit for surgery.

Familial pneumothorax

- Up to 10% of SP cases in some series have a positive family history. Need to consider potential familial cause such as Birt-Hogg-Dube syndrome, tuberous sclerosis complex, and connective tissue diseases.
- If suspected, CT imaging should be part of the standard work up and advice from specialists in this area should be considered.

ⓘ Complications

Re-expansion pulmonary oedema (RPO)

May occur as a complication of treatment for pneumothorax (up to 14%), especially in PSP present for some time before treatment. Higher incidence in large pneumothoraces and younger patients. Mechanism unknown but may be related to capillary damage and leak in the re-expanding lung. Reperfusion injury with free radical formation may also play a significant role.

Clinical manifestations

- Cough.
- Breathlessness.
- Chest tightness.

Management

- Observation: usually resolves within 24–48 hours.
- Avoid suction early in the treatment of PSP.

Surgical/subcutaneous emphysema

Definition

Air escaping into the subcutaneous tissues from a pneumothorax.

Mechanism

Air escapes under pleural pressure via a connection between the pneumothorax and the subcutaneous tissues, usually a complication of chest drain insertion. May occur if:

- Chest drain is non-functioning (kinked, mispositioned, clamped).
- Large air leak (insufficient drainage, especially COPD).

The patient

- Feel for 'crackles' as you compress the skin.
- Usually occurs around drain insertion site initially but may track to arms, face, and contralateral chest wall.
- Occasionally may be life-threatening (respiratory compromise due to upper airway compression). Look for facial involvement and/or voice change (laryngeal emphysema).

Management

Normally self-resolving and of cosmetic importance only. High-flow oxygen (increases rate of resolution) can be used unless the patient is known to retain CO_2. If evidence of upper airway involvement:

- Specialist referral as soon as possible.
- High-flow oxygen.
- Second/larger bore chest drain.

Tracheostomy is rarely required.

Chapter 28

Pulmonary embolism

Introduction

Pulmonary embolism (PE) can present with numerous non-specific symptoms and signs and hence mimics several other clinical conditions.

The annual incidence in the UK of PE is approximately 39–115 cases in 100 000. Half occur in hospitalised patients, with a quarter having clear risk factors and the remainder being idiopathic. Most hospitals will have their own protocol for investigation; some still use ventilation–perfusion scintigraphy if they have onsite facilities, but almost all now use CT pulmonary angiography (CTPA) as their first-line investigation.

This chapter outlines a practical strategy for the diagnosis and management of PE, including when to suspect it, associated clinical features, the key importance of pre-test probabilities, and the controversies around treatment.

PE is subdivided into massive PE and submassive PE according to the degree of haemodynamic compromise. Massive PE causes a systolic BP <90 mmHg (or fall >40 mmHg) for >15 minutes.

Risk factors

Major risk factors (relative risk 5–20)

- **Surgery:** especially major abdominal/pelvic, hip/knee replacement, post-operative intensive care.
- **Obstetrics:** pregnancy, caesarean section, post-delivery.
- **Lower limb fractures** and varicose veins.
- **Malignancy.**
- **Immobilisation:** institutionalisation.
- **Previous venous thromboembolism.**

Minor risk factors (relative risk 2–4)

- Cardiovascular: congenital heart disease, CCF, hypertension, superficial thrombophlebitis, indwelling central access.
- Oestrogens: oral contraception and hormone replacement therapy.
- COPD.
- Thrombophilia.
- Long-distance travel.
- Neurological disorders.
- Obesity.
- Chronic disease, e.g. dialysis, vasculitidies especially Behçet's.

Clinical probability

Before ordering any specific investigations for PE (including D-dimer) a clinical probability must be determined. Essentially all strategies for investigation rely on this, and if it is not consciously done then the pathway to exclusion or confirmation becomes unclear.

Scoring for pre-test probability: Wells' Criteria

The most widely used pre-test probability prediction tool in the UK is Wells' Criteria (Table 28.1)

- Score <2.0 considered low probability.
- Score 2.0–6.0 considered intermediate probability.
- Score >6.0 considered high probability.

Table 28.1 Well's Criteria

Clinically suspected DVT	**3.0**
PE at least as likely or more likely than alternative diagnosis	**3.0**
Pulse rate >100	**1.5**
Immobilisation >3 days	**1.5**
Surgery in the last 4 weeks	**1.5**
Previous VTE	**1.5**
Haemoptysis	**1.0**
Malignancy	**1.0**

Specific investigations once armed with pre-test probability

- High probability.
  - D-dimer is not helpful.
  - Proceed to CTPA (or VQ scan if CXR is normal and no cardiorespiratory disease—if available and CTPA contraindicated). If CTPA is good quality and negative then no further investigations are needed.
  - If VQ scan is non-diagnostic, proceed to CTPA.
  - In patients with coexisting clinical DVT, leg ultrasound as the initial imaging test may be sufficient.
- Intermediate probability.
  - D-dimer blood test—each laboratory has its own range.
  - If D-dimer above threshold proceed to CTPA (or VQ as above). If D-dimer is below threshold PE is excluded.
- Low probability.
  - D-dimer.
  - If above threshold, proceed to CTPA. If below threshold PE is excluded.

Submassive pulmonary embolism

► When to suspect submassive PE

Symptoms and signs in descending order of frequency from 70% .

- Dyspnoea.
- Tachypnoea.
- Pleuritic pain.
- Apprehension.
- Tachycardia.
- Cough.
- Haemoptysis.
- Leg pain.
- Clinical DVT (in only 10%).

Fever is common but completely non-specific (less likely if >38.9°C).

Examination findings

Tachypnoea and tachycardia should be noted. Occasionally a rub may be heard but these findings are neither sensitive nor specific.

General investigations

ECG

- Most common finding is sinus tachycardia.
- Non-specific ST and T wave changes are common.
- Right heart strain may be seen; the classic $S_1Q_3T_3$ is uncommon, but some features may be noted (Fig. 28.1).

CXR

- Most useful for demonstrating alternative diagnoses.
- Wedge-shaped classical pulmonary infarcts are rare and the oligaemic Westermark's sign is uncommon (➔ Chapter 55).

Other blood tests

- Arterial blood gases may show hypoxia and a raised A–a gradient.
- Raised inflammatory markers may suggest alternative diagnoses.
- D-dimer.
  - D-dimer is a breakdown product of fibrinolysis.
  - D-dimer is sensitive but non-specific for the presence of endovascular clot.
  - It is useful for its negative predictive value in low and intermediate probability venous thromboembolism, but has no useful positive predictive value.
  - This means that you should never investigate for a PE if the only finding is a raised D-dimer, as you are exposing the patient to the risks of the investigation.

Treatment of submassive pulmonary embolism

Therapeutic anticoagulation with either LMWH or DOAC should be started as soon as the diagnosis is suspected in high or intermediate probability patients and stopped if tests are negative. It can be withheld in low-risk patients until a D-dimer is available (although if immobile inpatients, consider prophylactic heparin). Dosing and preferred medication varies between locations—review your local hospital guidelines.

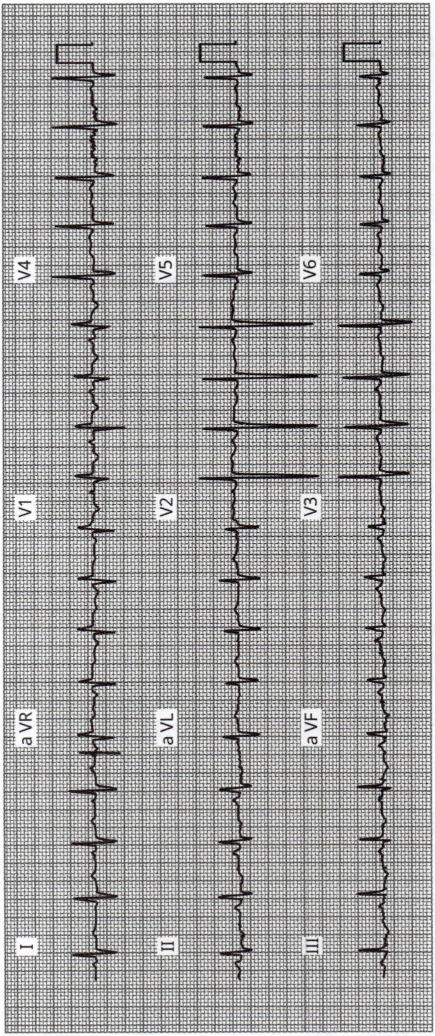

Fig. 28.1 ECG in a patient with multiple large PEs: note the S wave in I, inverted T waves in III, and the positive R in V1. However, there is no Q in lead III.

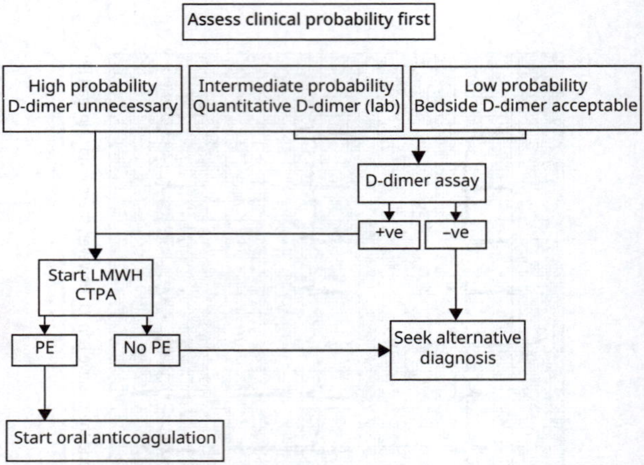

Fig. 28.2 Algorithm for management of submassive PE.

Duration of treatment

- For short-term risks (e.g. immediately post-surgery) 4–6 weeks is sufficient.
- For a first idiopathic thrombus 3 months.
- For all others 6 months.
- Long-term anticoagulation is often recommended in recurrent DVT/PE especially without significant risk factors.

Key areas of caution

⚠ *Renal failure (creatinine clearance <30 ml/kg/minute).*

- Dose adjustments maybe needed and some DOACs may not be used. If concerns, discuss with pharmacist or local haematology team.
- Some centres may use LMWH acutely in conjunction with anti-Xa activity monitoring.

⚠ *Pregnancy*

- D-dimers are likely to be positive (however, are still useful if negative).
- LMWH dose should be given according to actual weight (not pre-pregnancy weight).
- There is evidence that 10–20% higher doses per kg are required.
- Ideally anti-Xa levels should be monitored.
- Switch to unfractionated heparin as delivery date approaches.
- Liaison with experts in obstetric medicine is advisable.

⚠ *Obese patients*

- Some DOACs are not licensed in obese patients. Discuss with pharmacy if concerns. LMWH or warfarin may be required.

Mechanical options

Some patients are such high risk for anticoagulation that it must be withheld, e.g.

- Pelvic fractures awaiting fixation.
- Recent intracranial or spinal haemorrhage or surgery.

If anticoagulation needs to be withheld for more than 24 hours then mechanical options should be considered in consultation with interventional radiology.

- Clot dispersion or fragmentation using pulmonary artery catheter devices.
- Use of inferior vena caval filters to prevent further embolisation. Subsequent anticoagulation will be necessary to prevent filter occlusion and filter removal is possible at a later stage in some patients (if an appropriate filter is used initially).

Massive pulmonary embolism

When to suspect massive pulmonary embolism

Massive PE is likely if all of the following are present.

- Collapse and/or hypotension.
- Hypoxia without other explanation.
- Engorged neck veins or markedly raised JVP.
- Right ventricular third sound (gallop).

Managing shock in massive pulmonary embolism (➔ Chapter 1)

- High-flow oxygen.
- IV access.
- Analgesia (caution with hypotension).
- Ideally CTPA should be obtained prior to IV thrombolysis—most centres now offer emergency CT scanning 24 hours a day. If the patient is too unstable or this is not available, this may not be possible and should not delay administration of treatment. CTPA may indicate whether RV strain is present.
- Bedside focused echocardiogram in competent hands may identify RV strain. Elevated cardiac biomarkers (e.g. Troponin, NT-proBNP) may also indicate RV strain.
- Fluid load may be helpful but be very cautious beyond 500 ml as it may worsen RV failure and the increased RV wall stress may worsen the perfusion of and hence contractility of the right heart.
- See Fig. 28.3 for use of thrombolysis and heparin.

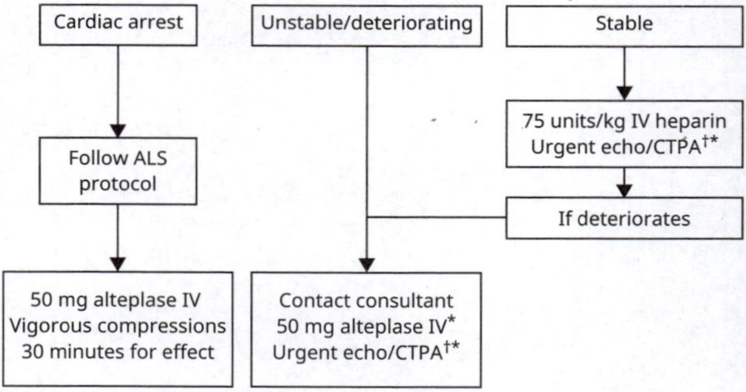

* If thrombolysis contraindicated because of high risk of bleeding, consider radiologically guided clot fragmentation or open thrombectomy if these facilities are available.
† Choice of echo or CTPA will depend upon expertise available and patient stability.

Fig. 28.3 Management algorithm for massive PE.

- If vasopressors are required then small boluses of metaraminol with institution of a noradrenaline infusion are the best option (➔ Chapter 1). Seek ICU support early if hypotension is significant and vasopressors are being considered.
- If central access is required make sure it is expert as accidental arterial puncture may prevent the subsequent use of thrombolysis.
- Avoid the subclavian route.
- Once PE has been confirmed, in stable patients give alteplase as 10 mg IV over 1–2 minutes followed by IV infusion of 90 mg. This may need to be discussed with a consultant depending on local guidelines.
- Thrombolysis can be followed by IV UFH infusion or can be commenced on S/C LMWH depending on local guidelines.

Treat in hospital or at home?

- With the widespread use of DOAC in PE, many centres are now moving towards ambulatory management in both suspected and confirmed PE in low-risk and stable patients.
- Risk-stratifying scores such as PESI and sPESI can be used as a tool to calculate which patients are appropriate for ambulatory pathways.
- PESI Class I and II and sPESI = 0 may be appropriate if the patient has no other risk factors such as being elderly, frail, confused, or having other comorbidities which might affect their ability to attend appointments or take their medication appropriately.
- It is worth checking your local guidelines to ascertain what pathways are available and what the criteria for ambulation are locally—these are usually accessible in the ED and the AMU.

Further investigation of patients following pulmonary embolism

- Testing for thrombophilia is only indicated if venous thrombo-embolism (VTE) is recurrent (without obvious major risk factors) or in those with VTE and a strong family history.
- If you feel thrombophilia screening might be helpful, discuss the patient with a haematologist before requesting the tests.
- If the patient is known to have a factor deficiency, discuss length of anticoagulation and preferred anticoagulant with a haematologist.
- Investigations for occult malignancy are only indicated in idiopathic VTE if symptoms, signs, or routine investigation raise clinical suspicion.

► Prevention of pulmonary emboli

Consider prophylaxis in all inpatients

- Peri-operative prophylaxis is routine practice in most hospitals.
- Medical patients are also at high risk because of immobility, particularly CCF, COPD, patients with chest drains inserted.
- Half of all PEs occur in hospitalised/institutionalised patients. Of those surviving the initial event, 7% die within 1 week, and 18% by 3 months *despite* standard treatment. Historical figures suggest a mortality of 30% without treatment.
- If chemical prophylaxis is contraindicated, patients should have TED stockings and automatic foot or calf compression pumps.

References and further reading

European Society of Cardiology (2019). Konstantinides SV, et al. ESC guidelines for the diagnosis and management of acute pulmonary embolism developed in collaboration with the European Respiratory Society (ERS): The Task Force for the diagnosis and management of acute pulmonary embolism of the European Society of Cardiology (ESC). *European Heart Journal*, **48**, 543–603. DOI: 10.1093/eurheartj/ehz405

British Thoracic Society (2018). Howard LSGE, Barden S, Condliffe R, et al. British Thoracic Society guideline for the initial outpatient management of pulmonary embolism. *Thorax*, **73**, ii1–ii29. Available online at: www.brit-thoracic.org.uk

Arachillage DJ, Mackillop L, Chandratheva A, Motawani J, MacCallum P, Laffan M (2022). Thrombophilia testing: a British Society for Haematology guideline. *Br J Haematol*, **198**, 443–458. Available online at: www.b-s-h.org.uk

Chapter 29

Pulmonary–renal syndromes

Introduction

The combination of new-onset respiratory signs, symptoms, and abnormal investigations together with acute renal dysfunction could indicate a 'pulmonary–renal syndrome'. Whilst renal dysfunction may follow on from systemic illness such as severe sepsis due to pneumonia, the term 'pulmonary–renal syndrome' is by convention taken to mean new alveolar haemorrhage and glomerulonephritis due to a systemic vasculitis.

Vasculitides are amongst the most interesting and challenging conditions which may present to the acute physician. Untreated, they have high mortality rates and therapy requires the use of high doses of immunosuppressant and often single or multi-organ support.

Classification

The pulmonary–renal syndromes are small vessel vasculitides and include the following.

- Granulomatosis with polyangiitis (GPA)
  - Upper airway problems and a positive c-ANCA/anti-PR3 are highly suggestive of GPA.
- Microscopic polyangiitis (MPA)
  - More associated with p-ANCA/anti-MPO. Hard to differentiate from GPA, especially as some MPA presentations (and vice versa GPA) will be positive for the alternate ANCA test.

The combination of immunofluorescence and anti-PR3/MPO testing increases sensitivity and specificity for the diagnosis of GPA and MPA to over 90% . Approximately 10% of GPA/MPA cases will be ANCA negative.

- Anti-GBM disease (Goodpasture's).
  - IgG antibodies attack antigens present in lung and glomeruli basement membranes resulting in glomerulonephritis and alveolar hemorrhage. Anti-GBM antibodies can be detected in blood.
- Eosinophilic granulomatosis with polyangiitis (EGPA).
  - The constellation of asthma, eosinophilic granulomatous airway inflammation, small vessel vasculitis, and peripheral blood eosinophilia >10% . May affect other organs; vasculitic neuropathy such as mononeuritis multiplex is common. ANCA positive in approximately 30–50% of cases, predominantly p-ANCA/anti-MPO positive.

History

Vasculitides are difficult to diagnose from the history alone. They should be suspected in patients who have been unwell for several weeks or months with non-specific symptoms. Patients have often been investigated and treated for other diseases. A 'vasculitic screen' will have been done as part of a search for the diagnosis.

Symptoms

- **Upper airway**: epistaxis, nasal congestion, sinusitis, mucosal ulceration, septal perforation, and laryngeal abnormality. In GPA upper airway symptoms are commonly the first noticed.
- **Respiratory**: haemoptysis due to small vessel vasculitis and alveolar haemorrhage is the classic symptom. Cough without haemoptysis, dyspnoea, pleuritic pain, and wheeze are also seen.
- **Renal**: frank haematuria is rare; oliguria may be seen as renal failure progresses.
- **Systemic**: malaise, lethargy, fever, arthralgia, anorexia, and weight loss are common.

Signs

- **Upper airway**: septal perforation and the classic 'saddle-shaped' nasal deformity point strongly towards GPA but are late signs.
- **Respiratory and renal**: commonly little specific to find.
- **Systemic**: low-grade pyrexia, vasculitic rash.

Investigations

Determining the diagnosis and exact type of vasculitis is important as it determines therapy. Routine laboratory tests and imaging will raise suspicion; specific diagnosis is made by a combination of autoantibody pattern and biopsy.

Urine

If renal involvement, positive dipstick test for blood and protein. Red cell casts seen on microscopy indicate active glomerulonephritis.

Blood

- Routine bloods, including FBC, U&Es, clotting.
- ESR/CRP.
- Creatine kinase.
- Blood cultures.
- Autoantibodies.
  - Antinuclear antibody (ANA), including anti-double-stranded DNA.
  - Antineutrophil cytoplasmic antibodies (ANCA): levels and type (c-ANCA/anti-PR3 or p-ANCA/anti-MPO).
  - Anti-glomerular basement membrane antibodies (anti-GBM).
- Other immunological tests including serum immunoglobulins and protein electrophoresis, complement levels, hepatitis B and C serology, HIV screen, and ASO titres may be helpful.

Chest radiograph

- Diffuse alveolar haemorrhage appears as bilateral patchy alveolar shadows. The differential includes infection or pulmonary oedema.
- GPA can produce a myriad of appearances (cavitation, pulmonary nodules, consolidation) and can mimic malignancy.

Arterial blood gases

- Hypoxaemia and hypocapnia result in an elevated A–a gradient due to alveolar haemorrhage.
- Elevated serum lactate can imply tissue hypoperfusion.

CT chest and sinuses

- Bony destruction of the sinuses can occur in GPA.
- Alveolar haemorrhage appears as diffuse ground glass change.
- In the acute setting CT thorax is of most use if an alternative cause of haemoptysis is considered.

Pulmonary function tests

- The textbook finding of an elevated corrected transfer factor (KCO) is good for monitoring response to therapy but is of little use acutely.

Biopsy

- Diagnosis confirmed by biopsy is strongly preferable. Site depends on nature of active disease and presentation. Commonly this is a renal biopsy but other extrapulmonary sites such as skin and peripheral nerves (e.g. in EGPA) are options. Lung biopsy may be performed in the absence of these extrapulmonary targets. Transbronchial biopsy at bronchoscopy is rarely diagnostic and thoracoscopic or open lung biopsy is required.
- When clinical features are typical and supported by autoantibody pattern (see classification above) a biopsy is occasionally unnecessary.

Management

For the on-call physician the management of pulmonary–renal syndromes should be as follows.

- Consider the diagnosis and its differentials.
- Assess the severity, in particular the level of organ dysfunction and need for critical care support.
- Ensure all the appropriate tests have been done.
- Liaise with an appropriate specialist for ongoing care. Nephrologists, respiratory physicians, or rheumatologists commonly manage these vasculitides.
- Initiate therapy if needed. Untreated GPA, MPA, and anti-GBM disease have a poor prognosis. Early initiation of immunosuppression can be both life- and organ-saving. If the suspicion is high enough, the correct tests have been sent off, and there is organ dysfunction, then immunosuppression is indicated.

Corticosteroids

- High-dose oral prednisolone, e.g. 1 mg/kg per day (up to 60–80 mg/day).
- High-dose IV methylprednisolone may be used for induction or if unwell, e.g. 0.5–1 g for 3 days, then change to oral prednisolone as above.
- In organ-/life-threatening presentations used in conjunction with other immunosuppressants. Usually, cyclophosphamide or rituximab.

Cyclophosphamide

In combination with high-dose corticosteroids. May be given IV or oral.

- Oral cyclophosphamide, e.g. 2 mg/kg/day up to 200 mg/day.
- IV cyclophosphamide, e.g. 15 mg/kg every 2 weeks for 3 doses and then every 3 weeks for 3–6 months.

Rituximab

May be used as an alternative to cyclophosphamide in combination with high-dose corticosteroids.

- IV rituximab, e.g. 375 mg/m^2 weekly for 4 weeks.

Plasmapheresis/plasma exchange

- May be used as an adjuvant therapy for those with severe renal failure or other life-threatening clinical manifestations such as pulmonary haemorrhage.
- Can remove circulating anti-GBM antibodies and has a role in anti-GBM disease or GPA/MPA with anti-GBM antibodies.
- Clinical practice may vary and requires the involvement of haematology, nephrology, or critical care teams.

Patients remain under long-term specialist management as immunosuppression is required long term and disease relapses can occur.

Further reading

Oxford Handbook of Respiratory Medicine chapter 50.

Part 4

Chronic respiratory conditions

Chapter 30

Bronchiectasis

ⓘ Introduction

Bronchiectasis manifests as a persistent dilation of the bronchi caused by permanent damage to their elastic and muscular structures due to ongoing inflammation. This dilation leads to inadequate clearance of mucus, consequently fostering recurring or persistent bacterial infections. The condition may present either as localised or widespread. In 40% of cases, a cause remains unidentified and the condition is labelled idiopathic. Bronchiectasis is estimated to affect around 1 in every 100 adults in the UK. Management is focused on treatment of the underlying cause, sputum clearance, infection prevention and prompt antibiotic treatment when exacerbations develop to minimise further permanent damage.

Diagnosis

Suspect bronchiectasis in patients with a persistent chronic cough (usually productive), shortness of breath, or persistent recurrent infections and consider underlying conditions that would put them at increased risk.

Investigations

- Baseline CXR during clinically stable disease
- CT chest to confirm diagnosis:
  - One or more of broncho-arterial ratio >1, lack of tapering, airway visibility within 1 cm of costal pleural surface or touching mediastinal pleura.
  - Bronchial wall thickening, mucous impaction, and mosaic attenuation in expiration are indirect signs.
- Check FBC, LFTs, serum total IgE, and assessment of sensitisation to *Aspergillus fumigatus* (via skin prick test or specific IgE), immunoglobulins, functional antibodies (if low vaccinate and recheck 4–8/52 later), HIV serology.
- Consider cystic fibrosis (CF) and primary ciliary dyskinesia (PCD) testing if suspected.
- Sputum cultures including routine and mycobacterial (TB and NTM).
- Pulmonary function tests (obstructive or normal usually).
- ECG.
- Depending on the history, more tests might be needed to identify the underlying cause based on history, such as RF, anti-CCP, ANCA, alpha-1-antitrypsin, protein electrophoresis.
- Bronchoscopy might be useful in cases of local disease (possibility of FB) or for diagnostic purposes if the patient is not expectorating.

Long-term treatment points

- *Haemophilus influenzae* is the most identified colonising bacterium (20–40%), followed by *Pseudomonas aeruginosa* (10–30%), *Moraxella catarrhalis*, *Streptococcus pneumoniae*, *Staphylococcus aureus*, and *Enterobacteriaceae*.
- Use the bronchiectasis severity index (BSI) to help guide management.
- Management includes:
  - Treatment of the underlying cause when possible.
  - Treatment of all co-existing comorbidities.
  - Chest clearance techniques, such as daily chest physiotherapy and mucolytics.

    - Nutritional support.
    - Prompt antibiotics for exacerbations.
    - Annual vaccinations.
    - Regular sputum cultures.
    - Pulmonary rehabilitation.
    - Clear self-management plans.
    - In some cases—when exacerbating three or more times a year despite optimal management—prophylactic antibiotics (e.g. azithromycin* or nebulised).
    - If continuing to exacerbate five or more times a year despite all the above, regular intravenous antibiotics every couple of months.
- In the deteriorating patient:
    - Ensure all the above are appropriately implemented.
    - Reassess pathogens and underlying causes, consider comorbidities (e.g. heart failure, PE).
    - Consider repeat CT imaging.
    - LTOT +/- NIV if criteria are met.
    - Consider surgery, transplantation, and end-of-life care.
- A new growth of *Pseudomonas aeruginosa* warrants an eradication attempt with oral ciprofloxacin or intravenous antipseudomonal β-lactam ± aminoglycoside for 2 weeks followed by a 3-month course of a nebulised antipseudomonal antibiotic.
- In patients colonised with *P. aeruginosa* needing prophylactic antibiotics consider inhaled antibiotics as the first-line.
- Inhalers are not indicated in bronchiectasis unless there is evidence of a co-existing lung disease such as asthma or COPD.

Exacerbation

- Symptoms: cough, dyspnoea, change in sputum (volume, colour, thickness), haemoptysis, pleuritic pain, lethargy, fever, malaise.
- Signs: airway secretions, wheeze, crackles, rubs.
- Radiological changes of infection.
- Investigations: FBC, U&Es, CRP, sputum for routine culture and mycobacteria, exclude pneumothorax, check total IgE and specifically to *aspergillus* (for ABPA, see below), check ABG if SaO_2 <94% or if there is ventilatory insufficiency.
- The choice of antibiotic is influenced by the colonising organism. The patient may have a self-management plan with a course of antibiotics ready to start at home.
- An effort should be made to send sputum cultures before any antibiotic treatment.
- For mild exacerbations, high-dose oral antibiotics should be given for 10–14 days. If a colonising organism is not known, treat with antibiotics as per CAP guidelines until sputum microbiology is available.
- For severe exacerbations, IV antibiotics chosen according to sputum microbiology should be given for 10–14 days. Consider oxygen or non-invasive ventilation.
- If colonised with *P. aeruginosa,* use ciprofloxacin 500–750 mg bd for mild exacerbations. If this treatment fails or the exacerbation is moderate/severe, then IV antibiotics should be administered.

- Anti-pseudomonal IV antibiotics should include a β-lactam (e.g. ceftazidime 1–2 g tds, meropenem 1–2 g tds, or piperacillin/tazobactam 4.5 gr tds) with or without an added aminoglycoside.
- Airway clearance with assistance from a physiotherapist. Urgent physiotherapist input is not needed out of hours unless the patient is very unwell.
- Consider bronchodilators before physiotherapy to treat wheezing and aid expectoration.

*NB: Prior to starting azithromycin, ensure LFTs have been checked, QTc is normal, NTM has been ruled out and the patient is counselled about hearing loss (might need audiogram).

Allergic bronchopulmonary aspergillosis (ABPA)

Definition

A complex hypersensitivity reaction in response to colonisation of the airways with *Aspergillus fumigatus*, occurs almost exclusively in patients with asthma and CF (it can also complicate non-CF bronchiectasis and COPD). Repeated episodes of inflammation, mucous impaction, and bronchial obstruction which can lead to bronchiectasis.

Diagnosis

Symptoms are usually of poorly controlled asthma with recurrent exacerbations. Dyspnoea, wheeze, thick sputum with occasionally brown plugs, and malaise are often present.

Diagnosis is based on clinical suspicion and the presence of the criteria below (the top 3 criteria have to be present):

- Presence of predisposing lung condition.
- Raised IgE against *Aspergillus fumigatus* or positive skin test.
- Total IgE >500 IU/ml.
- IgG against *Aspergillus fumigatus* >27 mg/L (if absent consider a higher total IgE cutoff).
- Consistent radiology.
- Eosinophilia, total count >500 cells/microL (can be historical, be cautious with possible concurrent corticosteroid use).

A similar syndrome can sometimes be caused by other fungi (allergic bronchopulmonary mycosis—ABPM). Two separate growths in sputum culture should raise the suspicion.

Treatment

- 0.5 mg/kg/day for 2–4 weeks, tapered and completed over 4 months of oral prednisolone.
- Oral itraconazole 200 mg bd is an alternative first choice or if corticosteroids are contraindicated.

References

- British Thoracic Society (BTS) bronchiectasis guidelines for adults (2018).
- NICE guidelines for adults (last revision 2024).
- Revised ISHAM-ABPA working group clinical practice guidelines for diagnosing, classifying and treating allergic bronchopulmonary aspergillosis/mycoses. ERJ 2024.
- https://www.nhs.uk/conditions/bronchiectasis/

Cystic fibrosis

ⓘ Introduction

Cystic fibrosis (CF) is an autosomal recessive condition that affects approximately 1 in 2500 live births in the UK. It is caused by a variety of mutations to the CF transmembrane regulator gene (*CFTR*), which encodes for a complex chloride channel. The defective function of CFTR protein results in viscous and sticky secretions.

CF usually manifests in the lungs as a cycle of inflammation and infection resulting in bronchiectasis and ultimately deteriorating lung health. Other multi-system consequences affect sinuses, pancreas, hepatobiliary system, kidneys, and reproductive system.

Most people with CF are diagnosed as children but latent diagnosis in adulthood is increasingly common and an important diagnosis not to miss. Half of people born with CF today are expected to live beyond 50 years of age and this is likely to rise further with the advent of new CFTR modulator therapies.

CF patients are usually managed by a multidisciplinary team at a regional CF centre and contact should be made with them (contact details available from www.cysticfibrosis.org.uk) as early as possible. Information from the patient and their notes will aid diagnosis and treatment plan.

Common treatment points

CFTR modulator therapy

CFTR modulatory therapy works by helping to correct the defective protein encoded by the CF-causing *CFTR* gene. Eligibility is based on genetic susceptibility to modulator therapy. The latest and now most prevalent iteration of CFTR modulator treatment is a triple therapy comprising of elexacaftor, tezacaftor, and ivacaftor (Kaftrio®) which is appropriate for 90% of the CF population. CFTR modulator therapy may have a multi-system impact beyond improving respiratory health and is an evolving area of understanding. It is important to note that not all people with CF are eligible for CFTR modulator therapy and some are intolerant. Although life expectancy for the CF population is expected to rise, people with CF still present unwell with complications of their condition.

Respiratory

Patients should be nursed in a side-room, if possible, to avoid cross-infection with different strains of *Pseudomonas aeruginosa* and other Gram-negative bacteria, particularly *Burkholderia cepacia*.

- 80% of adults are chronically colonised with *P.aeruginosa*.
- Antibiotic courses are given in higher doses and for longer than non-CF patients.
- Antibiotic treatment is usually 2 weeks in duration. Depending on clinical assessment these will be IV or oral.
- Choice of antibiotic for those colonised with *P.aeruginosa* is a clinical decision as in vitro resistance patterns do not always reflect clinical response.
- Azithromycin 250–500 mg od is often used for its anti-inflammatory properties in chronic mucoid *Pseudomonas* colonisation.
- Prednisolone ± itraconazole 200 mg bd may be used in ABPA.
- Mucolytic therapy in the form of Nebulised DNase (Pulmozyme®) and hypertonic saline is often used daily to reduce sputum viscosity and aid clearance.
- Physiotherapy-led airway clearance techniques are important as part of a strategy to aid secretion clearance.
- Aerosolised anti-pseudomonal antibiotics are used to reduce *P.aeruginosa* burden in the lungs. First-line treatment is usually with nebulised colistimethate sodium, for example Colomycin® 1–2 MU bd. Second-line options include nebulised tobramycin, for example Tobi® 300 mg bd in alternate months. These antibiotics are also available in alternative preparations. Additional anti-pseudomonal agents are available for those who fail to respond or are intolerant to initial strategies.
- Patients needing frequent IV antibiotics may have an implanted vascular access device (a central line terminating in a subcutaneous drum-shaped device) which is accessed by specially designed needles. These may become blocked or, rarely, infected.

Abdominal and extra-pulmonary

- Dietary supplements (including high-calorie drinks, nasogastric or PEG tube feeding) are often needed to maintain BMI >19.

- Vitamin supplements are taken by most patients, and bisphosphonates by some, because of malabsorption and a high risk of osteoporosis.
- Proton pump inhibitors are often taken to reduce oesophageal reflux.
- Creon or pancrease tablets are taken with meals and snacks to replace deficient pancreatic enzymes.
- Constipation is common and laxatives are frequently required. Common agents employed include lactulose and macrogols. Constipation is important to differentiate from DIOS (see below).
- Ursodeoxycholic acid may be taken to slow the rate of progression of CF-related liver disease.
- Slow-sodium 'salt tablets' are used (from four per day in the UK to 16 per day when in hot climates) because of excess salt loss in sweat. With CFTR modulator therapy treatment is less prevalent than previously.
- Insulin and oral hypoglycaemic agents are used for CF-related diabetes.

ⓘ Pulmonary exacerbations

Presentation

There are no universal criteria used to define a CF pulmonary exacerbation or its severity. A decision to treat a pulmonary exacerbation is a clinical judgement made on an individual patient basis. Common clinical features that may suggest a pulmonary exacerbation include:

- Increased cough.
- Increased sputum production and/or a change in appearance of expectorated sputum.
- Fever.
- Weight loss >1 kg or 5% of body weight associated with anorexia and decreased dietary intake or growth failure in an infant or child.
- School or work absenteeism (due to illness) in the previous week.
- Increased respiratory rate and/or work of breathing.
- New findings on chest examination (e.g. crackles and wheezes).
- Decreased exercise tolerance.
- Decrease in FEV_1 (of more than 10% from previous baseline study).
- Decrease in oxygen saturation.
- New radiographic signs in the chest.

Investigations

- Sputum for MC&S.
- Respiratory virus swab for PCR.
- CXR (assess for evidence of infection and to exclude pneumothorax).
- Check blood sugars (before and after meals).
- Check FBC, U&Es, LFTs, and CRP.
- Consider checking total IgE, aspergillus RAST, and anti-IgG (for ABPA, ➲ Chapter 28).
- Check ABG if SaO_2 <93% or if ventilatory insufficiency is suspected.

Treatment

- See Table 31.1 for common antibiotic choices.
- Chest physiotherapy at least daily (not needed out of hours unless the patient is very unwell).
- Nebulised mucolytic therapy such as hypertonic saline and DNase.
- Less severe exacerbations may be treated with oral antibiotics.
- More clinically severe exacerbations (or where oral antibiotics have failed) warrant IV antibiotics, administered via cannula or long line.
- Antibiotic choice depends on usual sputum microbiology and which antibiotics usually work (ask the patient). Local guidelines should be consulted as clinical practice will vary between local CF centres.
- In vitro sensitivities are often unhelpful for *P.aeruginosa* and *B.cepacia* complex. If no known chronic colonising bacteria, aim to treat *Haemophilus influenzae*, which is a common cause of exacerbation.
- Consideration should be given to stopping nebulised antibiotics when IV therapy is administered.
- If worsening despite antibiotics, check sputum results and antibiotic sensitivities, repeat sputum, and rule out haemoptysis, pneumothorax, ABPA, mucus plugging, and poor glycaemic control.

Table 31.1 Antibiotic choices for infective CF exacerbations

Bacterium	Oral antibiotics	IV antibiotics
H.influenzae	One of: Amoxicillin 0.5–1 g tds Co-amoxiclav Tetracycline Macrolide	One of: Amoxicillin 0.5–1 g tds Co-amoxiclav Third-generation cephalosporin
S.aureus	One of: Flucloxacillin 1–2 g qds (± fucidic acid) Macrolide Tetracycline Clindamycin	One of: Flucloxacillin 1–2 g qds Vancomycin Teicoplanin
P.aeruginosa	Ciprofloxacin 750 mg bd	One of: Ceftazidime 2 g tds Aztreonam 2 g tds Meropenem 1–2 g tds Piperacillin/tazobactam (Tazocin®) 4.5 g tds-qds PLUS one of: Tobramycin colistimethate sodium (2 MU tds) Fosfomycin
B.cepacia complex	One of: Doxycycline/minocycline Macrolide Co-trimoxazole Chloramphenicol	Combination of two or three antibiotics to be drawn from: Meropenem, Ceftazidime, Temocillin Aminoglycoside such as tobramycin (not colistimethate sodium) Co-trimoxazole

- Other treatment options include oxygen (beware CO_2 retention), nebulised bronchodilators, IV aminophylline or S/C terbutaline, oral or IV steroids (only if absolutely necessary), and escalation to higher level care for respiratory support.

Mucus plugging of the airways, ABPA

Should be treated as for bronchiectasis (➲ Chapter 30).

Haemoptysis and pneumothorax

➲ Chapters 6 and 27.

ⓘ Biochemical abnormalities

- Salt loss may cause dehydration and lethargy during hot weather. Replace salt and water orally or IV (0.9% saline) depending on severity.
- Hypomagnesaemia may cause lethargy. Replace with an infusion especially if also on an aminoglycoside (e.g. 20 mmol $MgSO_4$ in 500 ml saline over 6 hours). Oral magnesium glycerophosphate two tablets tds may help, but is very poorly absorbed.

ⓘ Distal intestinal obstruction syndrome (DIOS)

- Thickened secretions in the intestines may result in a subacute partial obstruction or acute obstruction.
- Clinical features of DIOS include constipation, abdominal pain, and vomiting. A palpable mass may be felt in the right iliac fossa.
- Plain abdominal X-ray often shows faecal loading in lower right quadrant and dilated small bowel loops with air fluid levels.
- Abdominal CT scan may help confirm diagnosis and rule out other pathology.
- Risk factors that predispose to DIOS include episodes of previous DIOS or meconium ileus, dehydration, poor glycaemic control, poorly controlled fat absorption, pancreatic insufficiency, and previous organ transplantation.
- Most people with CF and DIOS respond to medical management and surgical intervention should be avoided if possible.
- Mild (incomplete or pending) DIOS can be managed with oral rehydration and polyethylene glycol containing osmotic laxatives (e.g. Movicol®) or Gastrografin®.
- More severe presentations require IV hydration. Initial treatment is often with Gastrografin®. If no improvement Klean-Prep® may be given via nasogastric tube.

Further information

Oxford Handbook of Respiratory Medicine, chapter 24.

Notes on various elements of CF clinical care are available online at: http://www.cysticfibrosis.org.uk/about-us/resources-for-cf-professionals

Chapter 32

Interstitial lung disease

Introduction

Interstitial lung disease (ILD) is an umbrella term for over 200 conditions characterised by inflammation and fibrosis of the lung interstitium. Classification of this complex, heterogenous group is frequently debated and revised with terminology updated.

ILDs have broadly been organised into the following categories—idiopathic, exposure-related, autoimmune-related, sarcoidosis, ILDs with cysts or airspace filling and others. Each of these are generally subdivided into acute, subacute, and chronic causes.

Terminology can be confusing and often misused. For example usual interstitial pneumonia (UIP) is a radiological and/or pathological pattern seen in patients who have idiopathic pulmonary fibrosis (IPF). However, UIP and IPF are not synonymous with UIP pattern seen in a variety of conditions such as chronic hypersensitivity pneumonitis, collagen vascular disease, drug toxicity, and other causes. For more information on differentiating between specific ILD disease entities see the *Oxford Handbook of Respiratory Medicine*, chapter 31.

ⓘ Known idiopathic pulmonary fibrosis (IPF)

IPF is an aggressive condition causing progressive and permanent scarring with a median survival of around 3 to 5 years post-diagnosis if left untreated. It results in a restrictive lung impairment, with dyspnoea, cough, and hypoxia (particularly on exertion) being common findings.

Patients have variable disease progression and so outcome prediction is difficult. Factors such as smoking, environmental exposures, and gastro-oesophageal reflux disease have been shown to be associated with worse prognosis.

Objective measures of poor prognosis include a decrease in 6-minute walk test by more than 150 m within 4 years, decrease in forced vital capacity by more than 10% in 6 months, or reduction in diffusing capacity for carbon monoxide by more than 15% in 6 months.

Patients with IPF commonly present with worsening breathlessness. Common causes include, but are not restricted to, infection, pneumothorax, pulmonary embolism, heart failure, and pulmonary hypertension.

Acute Exacerbation of idiopathic pulmonary fibrosis (AEIPF)

Another important cause to recognise is the acute exacerbation of IPF (AEIPF) defined as an acute, clinically significant respiratory deterioration characterised by evidence of new widespread alveolar abnormality.

Previous definitions included a 30-day limit for the definition of acute but this has been reworded to 'typically less than one month.' Previous definitions also included the exclusion of infection but it is now recognised infection can cause direct lung injury and is a likely contributor to AEIPF. However, positive microbiology or virology in patients with AEIPF is low and comparable to patients with stable IPF. The difference appears to be an abnormally activated immune response in patients with AEIPF compared to stable IPF.

Assessment

- Bloods—There are no specific bloods required in the diagnosis of AEIPF but they do assist in ruling out other causes of breathlessness.
- CXR—Often carried out as the first investigation, it has more utility in ruling out other pathology, such as pneumothorax, than diagnosing AEIPF.
- HRCT—AEIPF patients will have background changes of their known IPF but new acute abnormalities such as increase ground glass opacities or consolidation, associated with alveolar damage, will also be present. Discussion with radiology to carry out the HRCT at the same time as CT pulmonary angiography will help to rule out pulmonary embolism.

Management

- Supportive—Provide oxygen and other supportive measures for symptomatic management. Discuss escalation planning early and communicate the high failure rate of invasive ventilation and how in most instances ward level care is most appropriate.
- VTE—These patients are high risk for venous thromboembolism and should have VTE prophylaxis where appropriate.
- Antibiotics—In the acute presentation infection can be difficult to rule out. Broad spectrum antibiotics are recommended for at least 7 days.

- Glucocorticoids—Steroids are commonly given in AEIPF. Prednisolone 1 mg/kg or methylprednisolone 1 g IV for 3 days followed by oral taper are common doses. There have been no specific clinical trials on the effectiveness of glucocorticoids in AEIPF and therefore evidence of benefit is uncertain.
- Antifibrotics—There is some evidence antifibrotic medication can reduce risk of developing AEIPF, but there is no guideline at this time that suggests starting antifibrotics for AEIPF.
- Lung transplant—Transplantation is a potential option for carefully selected patients. Clarify if the patient has already been assessed for suitability for transplant and inform the specialist team of the acute deterioration as this may expedite the need for surgery.

ⓘ Other idiopathic interstitial lung diseases

The majority of interstitial lung diseases, including non-specific interstitial pneumonia (NSIP), respiratory bronchiolitis-associated interstitial lung disease (RBILD), and lymphocytic interstitial pneumonitis (LIP), are generally seen and managed in outpatient chest clinics. Those conditions that are more likely to present acutely are briefly discussed below.

While quite different radiologically and pathologically, in general all these conditions are associated with a better prognosis than IPF and have a more favourable response to anti-inflammatory and/or immunosuppressive treatment. A similar approach to that described above should be adopted if these conditions present with respiratory symptoms as an emergency.

Cryptogenic organising pneumonia (COP)

- Presents with influenza-like illness, with cough, fever, malaise, and weight loss.
- <2 months of symptoms in 75% of cases.
- ESR and CRP raised.
- Multifocal and/or flitting consolidation on CXR.
- HRCT can show the extent of the disease and help rule out other causes.
- Differentiating from other conditions such as eosinophillic pneumonia can be difficult and bronchoalveolar lavage or transbronchial biopsy can assist diagnosis.
- 50% of cases are truly 'cryptogenic'. The remainder may be triggered by a variety of conditions, e.g. infection, connective tissue disorder, drug reaction, post-bone marrow or lung transplant, inflammatory bowel disease—these are known as secondary organising pneumonia
- Good response to steroids in 80% of cases.

Acute interstitial pneumonia (AIP)

- Previously known as Hamman–Rich syndrome.
- Presents with initial influenza-like illness, with cough, fever, malaise, and weight loss followed by rapidly progressive dyspnoea.
- <3 weeks of symptoms in most cases. Usually hypoxic at presentation.
- Extensive alveolar shadowing on CXR; costophrenic angles often spared.
- Diagnosed with HRCT, transbronchial biopsy, or lung biopsy.
- Radiological lesions are temporally uniform, i.e. suggest the triggering lung injury occurred at a single time point unlike UIP with lesions of different ages at different stages of inflammation and fibrosis.
- Treatment is with high-dose glucocorticoids or steroid sparing immunosuppression.
- In hospital mortality >50% and majority of survivors die within 6 months.

Progressive pulmonary fibrosis

Patients with ILD, other than IPF, with a known or unknown underlying diagnosis, can have radiological evidence of fibrosis. PPF is not a diagnosis, but rather describes patients with a more aggressive deterioration in the fibrotic component of their ILD. A wide variety of ILDs can manifest PPF, e.g. fibrotic hypersensitivity pneumonitis.

PPF is defined by the presence of at least two of the following:

- Worsening respiratory symptoms.
- Absolute decline in FVC by at least 5% predicted within 1 year or absolute decline in DLCO of at least 10% predicted within 1 year.
- Radiological evidence of progression of disease.

Patients who meet the criteria for PPF should be referred for urgent specialist review as they may meet the criteria for antifibrotic therapy (nintedanib or pirfenidone).

ⓘ Drug-induced interstitial lung disease

A huge spectrum of specific lung pathologies is encompassed in the above term. The best source of specific information about suspected drug-induced lung injury is www.pneumotox.com.

Difficulties arise in that frequently different potential manifestations may occur from the same drug (e.g. amiodarone can cause subacute cellular pneumonitis, organising pneumonia, and pulmonary fibrosis, to name but three effects), and the drug in question may have been discontinued some time before the onset of symptoms (examples of later presentations include nitrosoureas, radiotherapy, and amiodarone). However, the drug is usually still being taken at the time of presentation and has been taken for at least weeks and up to years.

Drugs most commonly causing ILD include the following:

- Amiodarone.
- Methotrexate.
- Cyclophosphamide.
- Gold.
- Penicillamine.
- Sulfasalazine.
- Nitrofurantoin.
- Cocaine.

There may be an associated peripheral blood eosinophilia.

Initial investigation and management is as for any other presentation of dyspnoea (➔ Chapter 2).

Hypersensitivity pneumonitis (HP)

Previously termed extrinsic allergic alveolitis (EAA), HP can present acutely within 4–8 hours of exposure to the relevant antigen (e.g. mouldy hay) (see the *Oxford Handbook of Respiratory Medicine*, chapter 30.

Clinical features

Characteristically dyspnoea, dry cough, and systemic upset (e.g. fever, arthralgia, myalgia, headache) with crackles (sometimes squeaks) on auscultation. Wheeze is absent.

Investigation and diagnosis

CXR may be normal (especially if significant time has elapsed from antigen exposure), although characteristically shows diffuse small (1–3 mm) nodules or infiltrates, often sparing the apices.

Routine bloods may show elevated inflammatory markers or neutrophilia. ABG may reveal hypoxaemia.

The most helpful clue to the diagnosis is a history of recurrent episodes of symptoms that resolve following cessation of antigen exposure with the above clinical findings.

Most cases will not require admission or specific treatment.

Where the clinical history is compatible with the diagnosis, and in the absence of significant systemic upset or significant hypoxia:

- Counsel the patient about avoiding further antigen exposure.
- Send off blood for serum precipitans analysis if known or available.
- Arrange chest clinic follow up (to ensure resolution of infiltrates or further investigation if needed).
- Arrange HRCT (characteristically shows patchy ground glass change and poorly defined nodules) and respiratory review. Corticosteroids may be needed. Atypical presentations will require further investigation (bronchoscopy with lavage and transbronchial lung biopsy or occasionally surgical lung biopsy) to exclude alternative pathology.

Chapter 33

Sarcoidosis

Introduction

Sarcoidosis is a multisystem granulomatous inflammatory disorder of unknown cause. It is a relatively rare condition (UK incidence 5–10 in 100 000) and so it is unusual for it to present in the acute medical setting.

Lymph node biopsy is carried out on over 90% of patients. More than 50% of these are from the chest with EBUS, with skin and palpable extra-thoracic lymph nodes the next most common sites. Biopsies have also been taken from heart, liver, and kidney reflecting the multisystem nature of the disease. Patients will often need concurrent care from multiple specialties depending on the sites affected.

Lofgren syndrome

5–10% of patients with sarcoidosis have their initial presentation as Lofgren syndrome—a combination of acute fever, arthralgia, erythema nodosum, and hilar lymphadenopathy on CXR. Treatment is supportive only, with the majority of patients having full recovery in 1–2 years. Differential diagnoses include acute tuberculosis and acute presentations of fungal infections. Erythema nodosum lesions should not be used as site of biopsy to differentiate as histology will show panniculitis regardless of the underlying aetiology, rather than granulomas associated with sarcoid.

Known diagnosis of sarcoidosis

Respiratory presentation

Causes of increased shortness of breath, on a background of sarcoid, are most commonly due to the following:

Flare of sarcoidosis

Comparison of CXR with earlier films is important. Both sarcoid and infection can cause an increase in shadowing on the CXR and discrimination between the two can be difficult, although dense consolidation (especially lobar) is unlikely to be sarcoid. Most patients will have spontaneous remission but for those with significant symptoms oral prednisolone can be considered. Most patients are given a moderate dose, such as 20 mg once a day, and response is assessed at 4 weeks followed by a rapid taper. For patients with more severe or progressive disease, a higher initial dose followed by a slower taper can be used. For these patients, a steroid-sparing agent such as methotrexate can be initiated in the clinic setting, under the review of a respiratory physician.

Infection

Treat as community-acquired infection. If the patient is on maintenance steroids, consider a transient increase in dose whilst unwell.

Pneumothorax

Occurs in cases of sarcoid with pulmonary fibrosis: treat as secondary pneumothorax (➔ Chapter 27).

Blood tests in sarcoidosis

The most common abnormality seen is lymphopenia. Between 15–25% of patients will have raised ESR, raised ACE, raised CRP or abnormal liver function. Less than 10% will have hypercalcaemia.

Non-respiratory presentations

- Hypercalcaemia.
- Skin: erythema nodosum (symptomatic treatment and NSAIDs), lupus pernio (see below), and cutaneous sarcoid.
- Cardiac sarcoidosis: most commonly presents with conduction defects. Therefore perform ECG on all sarcoid patients.
- Neurosarcoidosis: can present with any neurological symptom. Most common presentation is lower motor neuron facial palsy.
- Ocular sarcoidosis (sight-threatening): usually anterior uveitis. However episcleritis, scleritis, conjunctivitis, glaucoma, and retinal involvement can occur. Uveoparotid fever, also known as Heerfordt syndrome, patients present with anterior uveitis, parotid swelling, fever, and in some cases facial nerve palsy. Requires slit-lamp examination. Refer to ophthalmology.
- Renal sarcoidosis: rarely presents with acute renal failure.

Lupus Pernio

There are many cutaneous manifestations of sarcoidosis with up to 25% of patients displaying these at presentation. Lupus pernio is a distinct form which can be associated with severe granulomatous inflammation of the upper respiratory tract resulting in airway obstruction. It is characterised by erythematous, indurated, infiltrative plaques on the central face. Visual appearance of the erythema will vary with skin colour. For patients with severe disease or impending airway obstruction, expert specialist involvement should be sought and immunosuppression started. Glucocorticoids are commonly used but other agents such as Infliximab can be more effective.

Chapter 34

Respiratory conditions associated with connective tissue disorders

Introduction

Pulmonary complications are common in patients with connective tissue disorders (CTDs). They can be either specific respiratory conditions related to the CTD or side effects of medication used to treat the CTD, including opportunistic infection. When a rheumatological patient presents with acute respiratory symptoms, a number of disease-specific diagnoses should be considered.

ⓘ Specific respiratory conditions related to connective tissue diseases

These can predate symptoms of the CTD or develop later.

Respiratory conditions which might present acutely

Pleural effusion

- Common but often asymptomatic.
- Typically an exudate, often lymphocytic. Can mimic parapneumonic effusions with low pH and potential for loculations.
- Need to exclude other causes of effusion such as empyema and neoplasm (➲ Chapter 25 for approach to diagnosis and management of pleural effusion).
- The majority respond well to thoracentesis and 1 week of steroids.
- Persistent effusions require specialist input.

Acute pneumonitis

- Rare but high mortality rate.
- Presents with cough, dyspnoea, fever, and pleuritic chest pain.
- CXR shows infiltrates.
- Treatment is supportive: steroids and cytotoxics may be useful.

Organising pneumonia

- Presents with fever, dyspnoea, and consolidation on CXR, which may be multifocal and/or flitting.
- Raised inflammatory markers.
- Mimics bacterial pneumonia but no response to antibiotics.
- Good response to steroids in >80% of cases.

Pulmonary vasculitis

- Rare in CTD; more commonly associated with pulmonary–renal syndromes (➲ Chapter 29).
- Can present with alveolar haemorrhage and haemoptysis.
- Treat with high-dose steroids and/or cytotoxics.
- Plasma exchange may be useful.

Chronic respiratory conditions

Pulmonary fibrosis

- Most common respiratory problem associated with CTD, especially rheumatoid arthritis (UIP pattern usual) and systemic sclerosis (NSIP pattern usual). For further details, see the *Oxford Handbook of Respiratory Medicine*, chapter 31.
- Slowly progressive dyspnoea; bibasal fine inspiratory crackles.
- PFTs show a restrictive picture and reduced transfer factor.

Bronchiectasis

- Common; 30% of rheumatoid arthritis patients have HRCT evidence of bronchiectasis.
- More common in female seropositive patients.
- Diagnosis and management as for idiopathic bronchiectasis (➲ Chapter 30).

Pulmonary nodules

- Usually asymptomatic.
- May be seen as coincidental CXR finding in approximately 1% of patients with RA.
- Usually subpleural and can be up to several centimetres in diameter.
- Rarely cavitate; may cause haemoptysis and abscess formation.
- Cannot be differentiated from bronchial carcinoma on plain CXR (usually need CT thorax and biopsy).

Pulmonary hypertension

- Can develop secondary to pulmonary fibrosis.
- Systemic sclerosis can cause isolated pulmonary hypertension pathophysiologically similar to pulmonary arterial hypertension (PAH) (➔ Chapter 35).
- Presents with dyspnoea and features of right heart failure.
- Diagnosis is with echocardiography.
- Treatment is as for PAH but has better prognosis.

Obliterative bronchiolitis

- Rare complication.
- Presents with dyspnoea and hyperinflated lungs due to progressive irreversible airflow obstruction.
- Treat with trial of steroids but often ineffective.

ⓘ Specific respiratory conditions related to drugs used for connective tissue diseases

Methotrexate-induced pneumonitis

- Can occur in up to 1% of rheumatoid arthritis patients commencing methotrexate.
- Usually occurs within the first 6 months of therapy but can be seen within the first year.
- Symptoms are non-specific with cough and dyspnoea. Fever and crackles in 45%.
- CXR shows bilateral, predominantly basal, interstitial infiltrates. HRCT thorax demonstrates ground glass change with no zonal predilection. Diagnosis is difficult as there is a large overlap with hypersensitivity pneumonitis and rheumatoid arthritis-related fibrotic ILD.
- Stop methotrexate and discuss case with respiratory specialist as differential diagnosis includes opportunistic infection and bronchoscopy may be required.
- High-dose corticosteroids (60 mg/day) may be beneficial.

Leflunomide-induced pneumonitis

- Can occur within the first 4 to 6 months of starting treatment.
- Patients usually have previous exposure to methotrexate or underlying interstitial lung disease.
- High mortality (especially if patient previously had methotrexate-induced pneumonitis).

Rituximab

- Can occur weeks to months following last drug infusion. Peak incidence after fourth infusion.
- Can result in severe hypersensitivity reaction leading to death.
- Normally treated with cessation of rituximab and commencing IV methylprednisolone followed by slow taper of oral corticosteroid.

Anti-TNF therapy (etanercept, infliximab, adalimumab)

- Limited evidence suggesting association with anti-TNF therapy and the development of pulmonary nodules, granuloma, or progression of ILD.
- Features may simply be related to underlying connective tissue disease and not related to therapy although extra-pulmonary symptoms seem to improve.
- Further research is needed.

Gold

- Can cause fever and dyspnoea with pulmonary infiltrates on CXR and CT.
- Treatment: stop the drug and start steroids. Usually reversible.

Penicillamine

Can cause obliterative bronchiolitis, hypersensitivity pneumonitis, and pulmonary–renal syndrome with alveolar haemorrhage.

ⓘ Opportunistic pulmonary infection

- Patient may be immunosuppressed by drugs or by the underlying disease.
- Often presents with non-specific symptoms of low-grade fever, cough, and dyspnoea.
- Any opportunistic organism may be involved, including TB, PCP, fungi, and CMV.
- ➲ Chapter 13 for details of assessment and management.

Chapter 35

Pulmonary hypertension

Introduction

Pulmonary hypertension (PH) is classified into categories sharing similarities in pathophysiological mechanisms, clinical presentation, and therapeutic options. (WHO classification, see Table 35.1.)

Table 35.1 Classification and causes of pulmonary hypertension

► Pulmonary arterial hypertension (PAH)
1.1 Idiopathic PAH
1.2 Heritable PAH
1.3 Drug- and toxin-induced PAH
1.4 PAH associated with:
1.4.1 Connective tissue disease
1.4.2 HIV infection
1.4.3 Portal hypertension
1.4.4 Congenital heart disease
1.4.5 Schistosomiasis
1.5 PAH long-term responders to calcium channel blockers
1.6 PAH with overt features of venous/capillaries (PVOD/PCH) involvement
1.7 Persistent PH of the newborn syndrome
► PH due to left heart disease
2.1 PH due to heart failure with preserved LVEF
2.2 PH due to heart failure with reduced LVEF
2.3 Valvular heart disease
2.4 Congenital/acquired cardiovascular conditions leading to post-capillary PH
► PH due to lung diseases and/or hypoxia
3.1 Obstructive lung disease
3.2 Restrictive lung disease
3.3 Other lung disease with mixed restrictive/obstructive pattern
3.4 Hypoxia without lung disease
3.5 Developmental lung disorders
► PH due to pulmonary artery obstructions
4.1 Chronic thromboembolic PH (CTEPH)
4.2 Other pulmonary artery obstructions
► PH with unclear and/or multifactorial mechanisms
5.1 Haematological disorders
5.2 Systemic and metabolic disorders
5.3 Others

PH is most frequently seen as an acute admission either secondary to left heart disease or lung diseases/hypoxia; in such situations the clinical features will include those of the associated condition. PH outside these conditions is rare; this chapter will give a brief summary of clinical findings in this situation. Detailed discussion on diagnosis and management is beyond the scope of this chapter (see the *Oxford Handbook of Respiratory Medicine*, chapter 38).

Definition

Pulmonary hypertension is defined as a mean pulmonary artery pressure >20 mmHg at rest.

Presentation

- Relatively non-specific. Often a delay in diagnosis of ~3 years.
- Exertional breathlessness most common symptom.
- Angina-type chest pain from right ventricular ischaemia.
- Exertional syncope.

Examination findings include:

- Low-volume pulse.
- Elevated JVP.
- Right ventricular heave.
- Loud pulmonary component of the second heart sound.
- Pansystolic murmur (tricuspid regurgitation).
- Peripheral oedema.
- Low SaO_2.

Investigations

- ABG: low $PaCO_2$ and low PaO_2.
- ECG: right ventricular hypertrophy (high specificity but low sensitivity). RBBB with anterior ST abnormalities can occur. Prominent P waves suggestive of right atrial enlargement.
- CXR: enlarged proximal pulmonary arteries, enlarged right atrium and ventricle.
- Echocardiogram: enlarged right ventricle with septal flattening. The tricuspid regurgitant jet is used to estimate pulmonary artery pressure (operator dependent).
- Right heart catheterisation: confirms diagnosis. Allows the measurement of right heart pressure, cardiac output, and response to vasodilators.

Other investigations:

- Bloods including FBC, U&E, LFTs, ESR, autoimmune profile.
- Full pulmonary function tests.
- CTPA to look for thromboembolic disease.
- HRCT chest to look for interstitial lung disease.

Management

Once the diagnosis is made, referral to a specialist centre is required to coordinate chronic management of this condition. Patients with PAH and CTEPH should be considered for tertiary referral if appropriate for specialist intervention.

General management

- Anticoagulation: Many patients with pulmonary hypertension are at risk of venous thromboembolism and anticoagulation can be considered on a patient-by-patient basis.
- Oxygen: patient may be hypoxaemic due to a combination of reduced cardiac output and ventilation/perfusion mismatch.
- Diuretics: may be useful for treatment of oedema but may reduce preload.
- Graded exercise activities: patients should be encouraged to be active within symptom limits and supported with exercise programmes when stable.
- Vasodilator therapy: patients assessed during right heart catheterisation. High-dose calcium-channel blockers such as nifedipine (80 mg/day) and diltiazem (360 mg/day) used. Less than 10% of patients benefit.
- Prostacyclins: Infusions, oral and inhaled preparations of prostacyclin analogues or prostacyclin receptor agonists are available.
- Endothelin receptor antagonists.
- Phosphodiesterase 5 inhibitors such as sildenafil and tadalafil.
- Guanylate cyclase stimulator, e.g. riociguat is only class with license for Group IV PH, e.g. CTEPH.

Several surgical options can be considered, including heart lung transplant (see the *Oxford Handbook of Respiratory Medicine*, chapter 56).

End-of-life care

To improve symptoms of breathlessness, fatigue, and peripheral oedema (➲ Chapter 16).

Chapter 36

Respiratory problems in neuromuscular disease

Introduction

For the respiratory system to work both the oxygenation and ventilation of the lungs needs to work. Table 36.1 describes a variety of neuromuscular disorders that can affect the ventilatory pump at different sites. Most of these disorders result in respiratory muscle weakness or reduced efficacy of the diaphragm, which results in alveolar hypoventilation and impaired cough. Patients with known neuromuscular disease may present acutely with a presentation related to their underlying neuromuscular disease (such as infection) or occasionally in end-stage ventilatory failure.

Table 36.1 Acute and chronic neuromuscular disorders that cause ventilatory failure

Level of lesion	Acute disorders	Chronic disorders
Central nervous system	Head and spinal cord injury Stroke Tetanus	Multiple sclerosis Parkinson's disease Shy–Drager syndrome
Anterior horn cells	Poliomyelitis Rabies Encephalomyelitis	Amyotrophic lateral sclerosis Muscular atrophies Post poliomyelitis
Peripheral nerves	Guillain–Barré syndrome Critical illness neuropathy Diphtheria Herpes zoster Phrenic nerve injury Metabolic causes	Hereditary neuropathies
Neuromuscular junction	Botulism Organophosphate poisoning Snake bite	Myasthenia gravis Lambert–Eaton syndrome
Muscles	Corticosteroid myopathy Electrolyte disorders	Muscular dystrophies Myotonic dystrophy Acid maltase deficiency Mitochondrial myopathies Inflammatory myopathies

Assessment

Features to note from the history that suggest chronic ventilatory insufficiency

- Dyspnoea (this may be masked in patients with limb weakness).
- Early morning headaches and daytime sleepiness: due to nocturnal hypoventilation. Can develop before daytime respiratory failure.
- Orthopnoea (a feature of bilateral diaphragmatic paralysis).
- Ankle oedema due to cor pulmonale.
- Known neuromuscular diagnosis (e.g. Duchenne muscular dystrophy) or symptoms suggestive of an underlying diagnosis, such as limb weakness/swallowing difficulties.

Examination

- Chest examination may show rapid and shallow breathing with poor expansion and use of accessory muscles.
- Detailed neurological and muscular examination should be performed.
- Diaphragmatic weakness should be assessed in the supine position: results in an increase in respiratory rate; use of extrathoracic muscles and abdominal paradox may be seen.
- Look for other associated problems such as pneumonia and pleural effusion.

Acute investigations

- CXR: useful in looking for specific chest problems such as pneumonia or effusion. May show raised diaphragm suggesting diaphragmatic paralysis or right basal consolidation suggestive of aspiration.
- ABGs: the hallmarks of significant respiratory weakness are hypercapnia and hypoxaemia. Hypercapnia is a late sign and develops when respiratory muscle strength is reduced to <30% of predicted. Calculating the A–a gradient is often useful to exclude significant pulmonary disease (➔ Chapter 50).
- Spirometry: vital capacity (VC) is reduced but not sensitive for neuromuscular disease. Serial testing of VC may be useful to assess for disease progression. Diaphragmatic weakness may be suggested by a 15% decrease in the VC on moving from upright to supine.

Specialist investigations

- Nocturnal oximetry: nocturnal desaturation is an early feature of ventilatory failure.
- Respiratory muscle function: can be assessed in a number of ways but is more specialised. Includes mouth pressures, sniff nasal inspiratory pressure, sniff transdiaphragmatic pressure, and phrenic nerve stimulation.

Treatment

Acute presentation

- This depends on the underlying neurological condition and whether the patient is already in end-stage disease.
- Treat any underlying respiratory problem, most commonly bronchopneumonia.
- Oxygen therapy is vital, but keep an eye on ABGs for worsening hypercapnia and acidosis.
- Note: In patients with neuromuscular disease—evidence of hypoventilation such as hypercapnia is sufficient to consider ventilation. This depends on the patient's presentation and neuromuscular disease but keep in mind acidosis is not always required to initiate non-invasive or invasive ventilation.
- Chest physiotherapy is important to clear secretions as cough reflex in these patients is often depressed.
- Avoid sedatives such as benzodiazepines and respiratory depressants such as opiates.
- Close liaison with ITU as patient may require NIV or invasive ventilation.
- Specific treatments may be helpful for some conditions such as myasthenia gravis and Guillain–Barré syndrome. Involve neurologist at early stage.
- Serial spirometry may be helpful in assessing deterioration of respiratory function.

Chronic respiratory failure and non-invasive ventilation

- Ventilation improves mortality and morbidity but does not alter the course of the neuromuscular disease.
- As the condition progresses may need daytime support.
- Need to involve patient and relatives about choice of ventilation as neuromuscular disease will continue to progress.
- Invasive ventilation via tracheostomy may be required in some patients with bulbar muscle weakness. This should usually happen with specialist input from respiratory and neurology teams.
- End-of-life issues and palliative care are important.

Chapter 37

Sickle cell disease

Introduction

Sickle cell disease is one of the most common inherited conditions in the world, which affects predominantly people from equatorial Africa but also those of Mediterranean, Indian, and Middle-Eastern descent. It is caused by a mutation in the gene encoding the beta-globin chain of haemoglobin and is recessively inherited. Sickle cell disease is a multi-organ disorder, occurring most commonly in the homozygous form (HbSS).

Pathogenesis

The abnormal haemoglobin polymerises when low blood oxygenation occurs, leading to the formation of long strands. This deforms the shape of red blood cells from flexible biconcave discs into rigid structures forming a sickle shape, which block capillaries causing vaso-occlusion. This vaso-occlusion occurs throughout the body and causes multi-organ damage.

Natural history

- In the UK, most children are diagnosed at birth by neonatal screening.
- In countries where there is no screening programme, presentation is usually from 6 months and above, after fetal haemoglobin levels fall.
- The clinical course and age of presentation is highly variable.
- The most common complications are shown below in Table 37.1.
- Pulmonary complications include:
  - Acute chest syndrome.
  - Chronic sickle lung disease.
  - Pulmonary hypertension.

Table 37.1 Common complications of sickle cell disease

Painful vaso-occlusive crisis
Acute chest syndrome
Avascular necrosis
Acute splenic or hepatic sequestration
Aplastic crisis
Priapism
Proliferative retinopathy
Stroke
Leg ulcers
Cholecystitis

Acute chest syndrome

▶▶ This is a medical emergency requiring early recognition to prevent respiratory failure.

- Treatment is with IV fluids, high-flow oxygen, and prompt, adequate pain relief.
- Broad-spectrum antibiotics, including cover for atypical organisms, are often given as it can be difficult to exclude infection.
- Close monitoring is required with early involvement of critical care.
- Severe hypoxia is a predictor of severity and outcome.
- Involve a haematologist early as simple or exchange transfusion may be required.
- Bronchodilators and incentive spirometry may be of benefit.
- Venous thromboembolism prophylaxis is important, treatment dose anticoagulation is not routinely required unless there is clinical suspicion of pulmonary embolism.

Chronic sickle lung disease

Chronic sickle lung disease occurs secondary to an acquired vasculopathy as a result of recurrent damage to the small arterioles of the lung. A history of acute chest syndrome is an important predictor of chronic sickle lung disease, but it can happen in its absence.

Assessment

- Presents with progressive breathlessness.
- Can cause respiratory failure at end stage.
- CXR may be normal in the early stage but later shows features of fibrosis.
- HRCT is more sensitive and shows fibrosis.
- PFTs show features of restrictive lung disease with a decrease in lung volumes, the most sensitive early marker of chronic lung disease.
- All patients should be assessed for chronic lung disease at least annually with review of respiratory symptoms, respiratory examination, and oxygen saturations as minimum.

Management

- Management is difficult and there are no randomised trials to assess the most effective treatment strategies.
- Treatment options include home oxygen, hydroxycarbamide, transfusion therapy, and anticoagulation.

Pulmonary hypertension

This is common (~10% of adults with sickle cell disease) and an important cause of morbidity and mortality. Pathogenesis is thought to be due to haemolysis, releasing haemoglobin that acts as a nitric oxide scavenger, leading to vasoconstriction. Chronic hypoxia and thromboembolism may also contribute.

Patients are often asymptomatic until the late stages of disease.

Management

Patients should be referred to a tertiary pulmonary hypertension centre (➔ Chapter 35).

Chapter 38

Sleep-disordered breathing

Introduction

Sleep-disordered breathing encompasses two broad and sometimes overlapping groups: the first and largest is obstructive sleep apnoea/hypopnea syndrome (OSAHS), and the second is the nocturnal hypoventilatory disorders including obesity hypoventilation syndrome (OHS). Both require nocturnal respiratory support, usually via a nasal or face mask, although sometimes via a tracheostomy. The on-call acute physician may be consulted about patients who have sleep-disordered breathing and hence should be aware of the diagnoses and therapies.

Due to increased levels of obesity, sleep-disordered breathing conditions are becoming increasingly common.

Obstructive sleep apnoea

OSAHS is characterised by repeated upper airway occlusion during sleep. This leads to apnoeas (pauses in breathing) or hypopneas (underbreathing due to decreased airflow). Occlusions of the upper airway cause arterial hypoxaemia and hypercapnia, increasing respiratory effort against the occluded upper airway. The apnoea is terminated by an arousal from sleep to open the upper airway, allowing ventilation to continue. If this process is repeated many times an hour, sleep is fragmented, resulting in the characteristic symptom of OSAHS syndrome: excessive daytime somnolence.

OSAHS is very effectively treated by continuous positive airway pressure (CPAP) which is delivered by a tight-fitting nasal or face mask worn during sleep. The CPAP 'splints' open the upper airway throughout the respiratory cycle, preventing the cycle of occlusion, apnoea, and arousal. This leads to better quality sleep overnight.

Most patients with OSAHS do **not** have daytime type 2 respiratory failure and cor pulmonale. Patients with these signs may have an overlap syndrome such as obesity hypoventilation (see Table 38.1) or another respiratory problem such as COPD.

Table 38.1 Obesity hypoventilation syndrome

Obesity hypoventilation syndrome is a combination of:

- BMI above/or equal to 30 kg/m^2.
- Evidence of obstructive sleep apnoea or hypoventilation.
- Daytime hypercapnia $PaCO_2$ >/= 6.0 kPa.
- In the absence of any other causes of hypoventilation.

Treatment of OHS can be with either CPAP or NIV depending on the patient. NIV or CPAP should be continued overnight if these patients are admitted to hospital unless not safe to do so as the risk of decompensating into hypercapnic respiratory failure is present.

In a well person with OSA (not in ventilatory failure), CPAP is for control of daytime symptoms and can be safely omitted overnight if it is not practical to continue it.

Anaesthesia

Patients with OSA are at higher risk of anaesthetic complications. Ensure that the anaesthetist responsible for the patient is aware of the diagnosis.

- A 'difficult airway' may need a different induction technique.
- Anaesthetic, sedative, and opiate analgesic drugs cause muscle relaxation, increasing upper airway narrowing. They also blunt the respiratory drive and arousal mechanisms, worsening apnoeas.
- Extubation should be done when the patient is fully awake, preferably sitting up, with non-invasive CPAP available and appropriate staff on hand in case of a problem. Monitoring in recovery or on HDU maybe needed.

Respiratory

Presentation with cor pulmonale and ventilatory failure, i.e. 'decompensation' of OSA and overlap disorders, is discussed elsewhere (➲ Chapter 8). Therapy involves ensuring the use of CPAP or the introduction of NIV, diuretic therapy, and treating the cause of the deterioration.

Cardiovascular

CPAP is an effective therapy in acute cardiogenic pulmonary oedema in both OSA and non-OSA patients. Ensure that CPAP is continued in patients with OSA admitted with cardiogenic pulmonary oedema in addition to pharmacological therapy.

Nocturnal hypoventilation disorders

This encompasses a group of disorders in which pathology from brainstem to respiratory muscles results in the capacity of the respiratory pump being insufficient, with resultant ventilatory failure (➲ Chapter 36, Table 36.1). They are united by worsening hypoventilation overnight, especially during REM sleep; this results in arterial hypoxaemia and hypercapnia, although without the increased respiratory effort of OSA. The arousal from these episodes results in daytime sleepiness, morning headaches, cor pulmonale, and, as the disease progresses, chronic ventilatory failure develops.

- Part of the management of these conditions is long-term NIV. Varying levels of pressure support between inspiration and expiration augment tidal volume. This improves minute ventilation, resets central hypercapnic respiratory drive, rests the respiratory muscles, and therefore lowers $PaCO_2$. The daytime symptoms are ameliorated as the arousals are prevented and the blood gases are improved even during the day when NIV is not used.
- Patients using chronic ventilatory support should be under the care of a specialist physician (usually respiratory, but in some centres the service is run by a neurologist or anaesthetist).
- Support if needed or when specific questions arise is available from the specialist unit. As well as medical input there are usually physiotherapy or nurse specialists available during the day for practical issues.

Anaesthesia

Ideally, anaesthesia should be a carefully managed elective procedure. As in OSA the drugs used in anaesthesia suppress ventilatory drive.

Post-operative physiotherapy with early reintroduction of NIV is the key to avoiding respiratory complications. Elective admission to the ICU should be considered.

Respiratory

With ventilatory capacity diminished, many of these patients have limited reserve to withstand cardiorespiratory insults, such as pneumonia.

Omission of NIV is less well tolerated than omitting CPAP in OSA and therefore, if at all possible, should not be stopped.

- Worsening respiratory failure and cor pulmonale are the usual features of decompensation.
- Treatment requires addressing the cause of deterioration and continued NIV (➲ Chapters 8 and 44).
- Ventilator settings and entrained oxygen in the acute illness may need to be changed to account for changing lung mechanics.

Intensive care

The use of home ventilatory support should not automatically preclude ICU admission. Each case should be judged on its merits with careful consideration of the underlying diagnosis, reason for deterioration, premorbid state, and lung function, as well as the reason for ventilation, together with patient and family wishes.

Chapter 39

Known diagnosis of lung cancer

Introduction

Lung cancer is the most common cause of cancer death in the UK and therefore is likely to present to the acute clinician at some time. This chapter deals briefly with lung cancer itself; for more detailed information see the *Oxford Handbook of Respiratory Medicine*, chapter 32. Patients with a known diagnosis of lung cancer may present acutely with symptoms due to the primary problem of the lung cancer itself (which may or may not be with primarily respiratory symptoms), complications of treatment, or a respiratory presentation due to coexisting respiratory disease.

Although lung cancer treatments have advanced significantly recently, with the widespread usage of targeted therapies, stereotactic radiotherapy (SABR), and immunotherapy, as well as the more traditional surgery, chemotherapy, and radiotherapy, survival figures remain poor. Screening programmes are becoming more common throughout the UK and other Western countries due to the significantly improved survival for early-stage lung cancers. Those diagnosed with stage 1 lung cancer have a 65% 5-year survival rate, compared to a 5% 5-year survival rate for those diagnosed with stage 4 lung cancer.

Small cell lung cancer can be particularly aggressive—it has a 5-year survival rate for all stages of only 7% .

ⓘ Respiratory symptoms related to lung cancer

Clearly, all cardinal symptoms of respiratory disease (dyspnoea, cough, sputum, wheeze, haemoptysis, chest pain) can be present in patients with underlying lung cancer, but the most common reason for presenting as an emergency is increased dyspnoea. The reasons for presentation can be grouped into the following categories:

- Disease progression: pleural effusion, large airway obstruction, lobar collapse, SVCO, lymphangitis, pericardial effusion, diaphragmatic paralysis, chest wall infiltration.
- Complications of disease or its progression: pulmonary embolism, pneumonia (often occurring distal to the site of the airway obstruction by tumour), pneumothorax, anaemia.
- Coexisting respiratory pathology: COPD, asthma, pulmonary fibrosis.

One needs to keep an open mind as the presenting respiratory diagnosis may be *unrelated* to the underlying lung cancer (e.g. RLL pneumonia in a patient with localised tumour in the LUL).

Primarily non-respiratory symptoms related to lung cancer

Lung cancer most commonly metastasises to liver, bone, brain, and adrenals and may present with symptoms or signs related to this.

Remember the paraneoplastic syndromes.

The following is a brief non-exhaustive list of common presentations.

- Confusion or neurological deficit from brain metastases.
- Bone pain/pathological fracture: bony metastases.
- Leg weakness/back pain: spinal metastases. Neurological symptoms occur with spinal cord compression.
- Hyponatraemia (SIADH)—can present as confusion, seizures, or coma if severe.
- Hypokalaemia (ectopic ACTH).
- Hypercalcaemia (ectopic rPTH or bony metastases).
- Abdominal discomfort/swelling (liver metastases, ascites; consider constipation secondary to hypercalcaemia or opiate analgesics).
- DVT.

Attendance as a complication of therapy

Patients undergoing chemotherapy for both small-cell and non-small-cell lung cancer may present with complications of this treatment, particularly neutropaenic sepsis (treat as per hospital guidelines).

Following lung resection, risks include empyema, wound infection, and pulmonary embolism.

Pneumonitis following radiotherapy can cause clinical symptoms in 7–8% of patients (although radiographically more frequent, ~40%). This is much more frequent following radical rather than palliative radiotherapy and presents after 2–3 months, usually with a non-productive cough, dyspnoea, and/or fever.

Immunotherapy, although often well tolerated, can cause a multitude of autoimmune reactions including pneumonitis, skin reactions, myocarditis, colitis, hepatitis, and endocrinopathies such as thyroiditis or adrenal failure. The treatment is usually withholding the offending medication and suppressing inflammation with steroids/other immunosuppressants. Some of these reactions can be severe and life-threatening—if you suspect a significant immunotherapy reaction, an urgent acute oncology opinion should be sought for advice on how to manage this.

In certain centres, endobronchial treatment is performed for palliation of large airway obstruction by tumour, e.g. endobronchial diathermy, laser, or stenting. Complications include fever, infection, and bleeding. Stents can migrate and either block previously patent lobar bronchi or come to rest in the trachea, requiring removal.

ⓘ Presentation with unrelated illness

Although lung cancer survival overall is low (10–15% overall at 5 years), there are subgroups who, with appropriate treatment, can hope for a much better outlook. This must be borne in mind when making decisions about aggressive treatment (e.g. deciding on ITU admission) for other acute medical problems.

Assessment and evaluation

Important points in the history (old notes/clinic letters obviously valuable):

- Timing and nature of diagnosis.
- Known extent of disease on staging CT/PET.
- Specific anti-cancer treatments (including those planned).
- Prior local chest intervention (pleural aspiration/endobronchial intervention).
- Respiratory comorbidity.

In assessing the patient, other than the mandatory CXR, routine blood tests may provide helpful pointers as to the cause of presentation, e.g. high inflammatory markers in infection or coexisting problems such as anaemia or SIADH.

In the breathless patient with an unremarkable or unchanged CXR and little else to find, consider large airway obstruction or PE. Large airway obstruction is often missed in the patient with mild dyspnoea. Listen carefully close to the patient's mouth for stridor.

Consider pericardial effusion. Is there clinical evidence of tamponade, small QRS complexes on ECG? Has the heart enlarged on CXR?

Do not measure D-dimers; they are very non-specific and will be elevated in active cancer. If PE is suspected, request a CTPA.

An up-to-date CT scan is often needed to clarify the cause of increased or new symptoms if not readily apparent on the CXR or from routine investigations.

Management

This would be dictated by the suspected diagnosis and would generally not be any different to the non-lung cancer patient. Early discussion with the respiratory team is important.

Specific situations

Pleural effusion

If pleural malignancy is not known, a diagnostic/therapeutic tap is best first-line management where cytological results will affect management (e.g. previously suspected limited disease and radical treatment proposed; if initial cytology negative, thoracoscopy may be needed). If presenting in a patient with more advanced disease and causing significant symptoms, therapeutic pleural aspiration of up to 1.5 L would be reasonable in the first instance.

If known malignant effusion and patient is symptomatic and the effusion recurs, chest drain with talc pleurodesis, indwelling pleural catheter insertion, or medical thoracoscopy with talc poudrage could be considered depending on what is available locally, patient fitness, and preference. If the patient is very fit then video-assisted thoracoscopy (VATS) pleurectomy with talc poudrage should be considered.

Malignant large airway obstruction

Start dexamethasone (8 mg bd) and request an urgent CT scan (usually can wait until normal working hours). Refer to respiratory team for consideration of palliative radiotherapy ± endobronchial intervention.

Haemoptysis

➲ Chapter 6.

Part 5

Practical management issues

Airway management

Introduction

Partial or complete upper airway obstruction is a medical emergency that requires urgent intervention. There are many causes of upper airway obstruction, but it is mostly seen in those with reduced levels of consciousness for whatever reason. An early call for anaesthetic support is crucial but simple airway maneouvres and adjuncts may temporarily relieve the obstruction and provide stability whilst anaesthetic support is awaited and advanced airway equipment prepared.

The insertion of a supraglottic airway device (SGAD) is relatively straight forward and can be inserted in emergency scenarios to provide airway protection and ventilation. Tracheal intubation is the 'gold standard' for securing the airway. It facilitates positive pressure ventilation, prevents air leakage even with high inflation pressures, and protects the lungs from soiling with gastric contents or other material (e.g. blood). Can't intubate, can't oxygenate (CICO) after failed upper airway management is a life-threatening situation that requires emergency front of neck access (eFONA). The recommended technique is scalpel cricothyroidotomy using the 'scalpel-bougie-tube' technique.

Aims of airway management

- To relieve upper airway obstruction.
- To facilitate positive pressure ventilation.
- To protect respiratory tract from aspiration of gastric contents.

Upper airway obstruction

The upper airway stretches from the mouth and nose to the carina.

Level of obstruction

- Supraglottic (above vocal cords).
- Glottic (involving vocal cords).
- Infraglottic (below vocal cords).

Most sudden and acutely life-threatening obstructions are supraglottic.

Causes

Functional

- Central nervous system depression (e.g. cerebrovascular accident, traumatic brain injury, metabolic, alcohol).
- Peripheral nervous and neuromuscular dysfunction (e.g. recurrent laryngeal nerve palsy, laryngospasm, Guillain–Barré syndrome).

Mechanical

- Foreign body (including vomitus).
- Oedema.
- Infection.
- Haematoma.
- Trauma.
- Burns.
- Neoplasm.
- Congenital.

Clinical signs

In a conscious patient the diagnosis is often easy. In unconscious patients a high index of suspicion, adequate exposure of the patient, and careful examination are required. A brief history from witnesses, paramedics, etc. may lead to the cause.

Complete obstruction

- Silent.
- Unable to breathe or speak despite forceful respiratory effort.
- Tracheal tug and intercostal recession.
- Hand on throat.
- Agitation and distress.

⚠ Emergency! Unless treated immediately, the patient will likely die within minutes.

Partial obstruction

- Noisy.
- Inspiratory stridor, gurgling, choking.
- Paradoxical chest wall movement ('see-sawing').
- Tracheal tug and intercostal recession.

⚠ Emergency! Without prompt intervention the patient is at high risk of deteriorating rapidly into complete obstruction.

Simple airway manoeuvres and adjuncts

Upper airway obstruction is a commonly encountered emergency that can often be relieved by simple basic airway manoeuvres.

Many of these patients will require more advanced management such as the placement of a definitive airway (e.g. tracheal intubation). These procedures carry both a higher failure rate and significant complication risks and thus should only be performed by experienced practitioners. Therefore, it is vitally important to call for anaesthetic help early. The simple techniques described below may provide stability whilst anaesthetic support is awaited and advanced airway equipment prepared.

Airway manoeuvres

These are used to overcome upper airway obstruction and subsequently maintain airway patency.

Head tilt and chin lift

Extend the neck by placing one hand on the patient's forehead and tilting the head backwards whilst simultaneously using the fingers of the other hand to push the chin upwards, lifting the jaw. Avoid this technique in suspected cervical spine injury and use a jaw thrust instead.

Jaw thrust

Whilst anchoring the heel of your palms on the patient's cheekbones, place the tips of your fingers behind the angle of the jaw and pull forward. At the same time open the mouth with your thumbs.

Suction

A wide-bore sucker (e.g. Yankauer) can be used to clear the upper airway of gastric contents, blood, and saliva. It is best used in conjunction with a laryngoscope or tongue depressor to prevent pharyngeal trauma and bleeding. Conscious patients may gag and vomit.

Simple airway adjuncts

These simple pieces of equipment can overcome upper airway obstruction in patients with a reduced level of consciousness. They also facilitate suction of the airway and the administration of oxygen via a face mask.

Oropharyngeal airway (OPA)

This rigid curved plastic tube is easily inserted upside down with the curved side towards the tongue before being rotated 180 degrees once it has advanced as far as the soft palate. It is then pushed in further until the flanged end sits at the patient's lips. It will likely not be tolerated in conscious or semiconscious patients with an intact gag reflex. Its length equates to the vertical distance between the angle of the jaw and the patient's incisors with sizes 4 and 5 most used in adults.

Nasopharyngeal airway (NPA)

This is a soft plastic tube with a bevel at one end and a flange at the other. It is generally better tolerated than an OPA in the semi-conscious patient. Sizes 6–7 mm are suitable for most adults. The airway is lubricated with water-soluble jelly and the bevel end inserted into the nostril and gently advanced backwards in a pushing and twisting motion. Mucosal damage and bleeding are common. NPAs are relatively contraindicated in base-of-skull fractures. Its length equates to the distance between the tip of the nose and the tragus of the ear.

Supraglottic airway devices (SGADs)

SGADs are used electively in anaesthetic practice for simple low risk cases but given the relative simplicity of their insertion with minimal experience they can have a key role in emergencies as a rescue device or an alternative to tracheal intubation. The most-used SGADS are the laryngeal mask airway (LMA) which consists of a wide-bore tube and inflatable cuff and the I-gel which has a non-inflatable gel cuff. The cuff of both devices is positioned over the larynx creating a relative seal that allows for ventilation and reduces the risk of gastric aspiration in the unconscious patient. However, in cases of high airway resistance (e.g. severe asthma) or poor lung compliance the high inspiratory pressures may produce a significant leak, compromising ventilation and causing gastric inflation. Newer generations of these devices have integrated bite blocks and gastric ports to aspirate gastric contents.

LMA insertion

- Size 4 LMA if patient weight is 50–70 kg and size 5 if >70 kg.
- Test the cuff by fully inflating it and then fully deflate and apply water-soluble jelly to the outer part of the cuff.
- Standing behind the patient, open their mouth and extend their head to the sniffing position, unless a cervical spine injury is suspected when a jaw thrust can be used to aid insertion.
- Hold the LMA like a pen and insert it into the mouth with the black line on the tube facing the patient's nose and the opening pointing towards the patient's feet.
- Guiding the mask with your index finger, push upwards and backwards to allow it to slide along the hard palate. When it reaches the posterior pharyngeal wall push slightly downwards until resistance is felt.
- Inflate the cuff with air (usually 30 ml for size 4 and 40 ml for size 5). If placed correctly the LMA should slide out by about 1–2 cm.

I-gel insertion

- Size 3 if patient weight is 30–60 kg, 4 if 50–90 kg, and 5 if >90 kg.
- Lubricate the back and sides of the cuff with a water-soluble jelly.
- Standing behind the patient, open their mouth and extend their head to the sniffing position, unless a cervical spine injury is suspected when a jaw thrust can be used to aid insertion.
- With the I-gel cuff outlet facing the patient's chin, introduce the device tip into the mouth, directing towards the hard palate. Slide downwards and backwards along the hard palate until resistance is felt.
- A jaw thrust or slight rotation of the device may assist insertion.

Following SGAD insertion connect the device to a self-inflating bag with oxygen and inflate the chest. If placed correctly there should be minimal or no audible leak. Auscultate the chest to confirm air entry and secure the device in place. If unsuccessful or in doubt remove the SGAD and oxygenate with a face mask.

Tracheal intubation

This is the 'gold standard' for securing the airway. It facilitates positive pressure ventilation, prevents air leakage even with high inflation pressures, and protects the lungs from soiling with gastric contents or other material (e.g. blood).

However, tracheal intubation, especially in an emergency, can be very difficult and should only be undertaken by practitioners who have been appropriately trained. In inexperienced hands the risk of unrecognised misplacement of the tube is high and can result in hypoxia and death. In conscious or semiconscious patients an emergency anaesthetic is required, which poses its own significant risks.

❗If you are unfamiliar with tracheal intubation, call for expert help and oxygenate the patient using non-invasive techniques.

In the case of emergency intubations, a checklist or LocSSIP (local safety standards for invasive procedures) should be used to ensure adequacy of personnel and equipment as well as informing all team members of the plan in case of difficulty.

Predictors of difficulty

- High Mallampati score.
- Inability to protrude mandible.
- Limited mouth opening—Interincisor gap <3 cm.
- Reduced neck movement—Thyromental distance <7 cm.
- Obesity.
- Previous difficult intubation.

Equipment required as per pre-intubation checklist

- Cuffed tracheal tubes: size 7.0 (internal diameter in millimetres) for females and size 8.0 for males plus one size above and below.
- Syringe for cuff inflation.
- Laryngoscope: usually Macintosh (curved) size 3 or 4.
- Videolaryngoscope such as McGrath (now commonly used on first attempt).
- Water-soluble lubricating jelly.
- Magill's forceps.
- Gum elastic bougie.
- Tape or tie to secure tube in place.
- Stethoscope.
- Suction with Yankauer attachment.
- End-tidal CO_2 detector.
- Appropriate haemodynamic and respiratory monitoring.
- Breathing circuit (self-inflating bag or water circuit).
- Personal protective equipment (PPE).
- Difficult intubation trolley (location must be known and near-by).

Technique

- Position patient supine and flat with head in sniffing position (pillow under head and shoulders).
- Pre-oxygenate with high-flow oxygen and bag and mask.
- Anaesthetic drugs are administered as required.

- Cricoid pressure is applied by an assistant, usually an operating department practitioner (ODP), in patients at risk of pulmonary aspiration of gastric contents such as those not starved prior to emergency intubation. The assistant places their thumb and index finger onto the cricoid cartilage and applies a pressure of 30 N (3 kg) in an anteroposterior direction. Evidence for the use of cricoid pressure is very limited and thus the technique is not standard in most other countries.
- Standing behind the patient, hold the laryngoscope with your left hand and advance the blade along the right edge of the tongue into the pharynx. Place the tip of the blade into the vallecula between the root of the epiglottis and the base of the tongue.
- Lift the laryngoscope forwards and upwards (do not tilt or touch the incisors), which pulls the epiglottis up and brings the vocal cords into view.
- Insert the tube through the vocal cords so that the cuff is fully past the cords.
- Withdraw the laryngoscope and inflate the cuff.
- Confirm placement by auscultating breath sounds bilaterally and detection of end-tidal CO_2 on five consecutive breaths. Once confirmed the tube can be secured.
- If end-tidal CO_2 is not detected, then this is considered to be an oesophageal intubation and the tube should be removed immediately. The patient should be oxygenated and ventilated using a bag-mask and airway adjuncts until re-attempting intubation.
- A chest X-ray is performed post-intubation to confirm optimal endotracheal tube position, which is 2–3 cm above the carina.

Emergency front of neck access (eFONA)

The indication for eFONA access is the life-threatening situation of 'can't intubate, can't oxygenate' (CICO) after failed upper airway management (Fig. 40.1). There are three recognised techniques for establishing front of neck access: scalpel cricothyroidotomy, cannula cricothyroidotomy, and surgical tracheostomy. Scalpel cricothyroidotomy using the 'scalpel-bougie-tube' technique is currently recommended as first-line.

Scalpel cricothyroidotomy

Assemble a number 10 scalpel blade, a size 6.0 mm cuffed endotracheal tube, and a bougie.

- 100% oxygen is applied to the upper airway, the neck is fully extended, and adequate neuromuscular blockers administered.
- Laryngeal handshake performed to identify and palpate the cricothyroid membrane.
- Perform a transverse stab incision through the skin and membrane.
- Rotate the blade 90 degrees (sharp edge towards feet).
- Slide tip of bougie alongside of blade into the trachea.
- Insert a lubricated size 6.0 mm tracheal tube over the bougie into the trachea. Remove bougie and inflate the cuff.
- Ventilate with a self-inflating bag and confirm position with auscultation and end-tidal CO_2 detector before securing in place.

Cannula cricothyroidotomy

This technique is no longer recommended first-line due to its high risk of failure and complications. The lungs are inflated via a kink-resistant cannula inserted 45 degrees caudally through the cricothyroid membrane into the trachea. Exhalation is passive as air passes through the upper airway.

Narrow bore cricothyroidotomy requires a specialised high-pressure ventilation system such as transtracheal jet ventilation which has been associated with high rates of failure and barotrauma.

Large bore cricothyroidotomy can be performed using a guidewire technique which has the advantage of being compatible with conventional ventilation. However, again it has been shown to have high failure rates.

If performed, adequate time for exhalation must be allowed and if ventilation fails or surgical emphysema develops it should be converted to a scalpel cricothyroidotomy.

Emergency tracheostomy

An emergency percutaneous or surgical tracheostomy takes longer to perform than a scalpel cricothyroidotomy and requires both specialist equipment and an experienced operator.

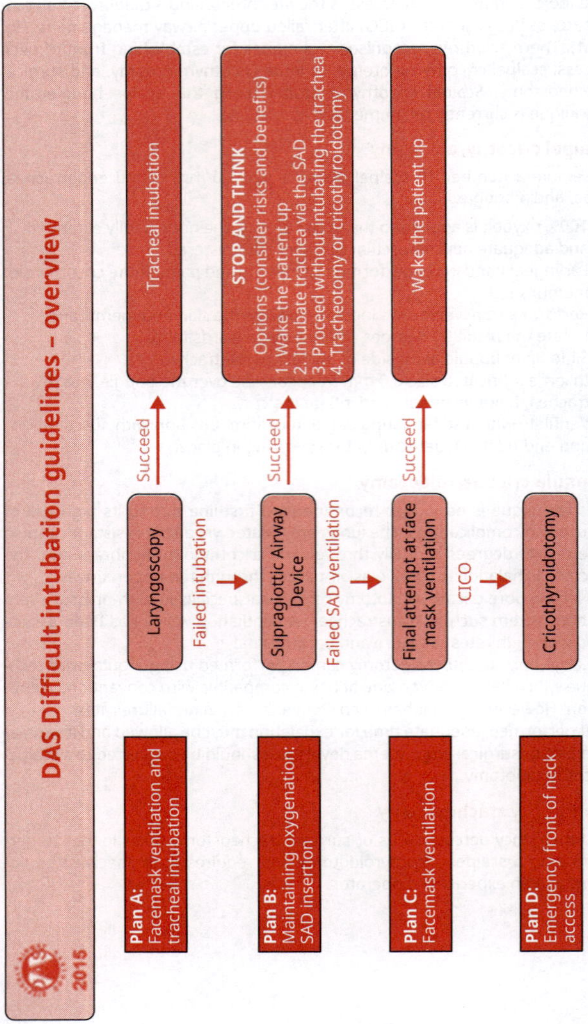

Fig. 40.1 Difficult Airway Society difficult intubation algorithm. Reproduced with kind permission from Difficult Airway Society (DAS).

Ventilation

If a patient is apnoeic or their respiration is inadequate, despite a patent airway, then ventilatory support should be provided.

Face mask ventilation

A face mask can be used in conjunction with simple airway maneouvres and adjuncts, such as an OPA and/or NPA, to optimise oxygenation if respiratory effort is adequate. In those with a reduced conscious level accompanied by sub-optimal respiratory effort or apnoeas a face mask can also be used to deliver ventilatory support via a self-inflating bag or breathing circuit. When manually ventilating one hand holds the mask onto the face with the thumbs whilst the fingers perform a jaw thrust and pull the face into the mask. The other hand can be used to compress the bag and ventilate the patient. A two-person technique allows one person to focus on opening the airway and maintaining a good seal around the face whilst the other delivers ventilation. This technique can reduce the risk of gastric inflation and improve the effectiveness of ventilation.

Initially, the patient should be ventilated with 100% oxygen, which can subsequently be weaned as required, at a rate of 12–16 breaths/minute. We aim to deliver tidal volumes of 6 ml/kg body weight, which commonly equates to 400–600 ml. Given that the volume of the bag is 2 L, we must be careful to only deliver roughly a quarter of the bag volume with any one breath to avoid barotrauma and gastric distension.

Mechanical ventilation

Evidence has shown that lung protective ventilation strategies such as those defined in the ARDSNET trial significantly improve mortality. Therefore, the recommendation is that mechanically ventilated patients receive tidal volumes equivalent to 6 ml/kg body weight and plateau pressures <30 cmH_2O.

Effects of ventilation on circulation

Positive-pressure ventilation has many effects on cardiovascular physiology, a few of which are described below.

As intrathoracic pressure increases, venous return and preload are reduced, leading to a fall in cardiac output. This response may be exaggerated in hypovolaemic patients. However, in patients with cardiac pulmonary oedema, the reduction in preload and afterload may improve cardiac function.

Other effects are due to changes in partial pressure of CO_2. Hypocapnia causes an increase in systemic vascular resistance, afterload, and myocardial workload. This may lead to a fall in cardiac output and a reduction in blood flow to vital organs. Hypercapnia causes vasodilatation and stimulates sympathetic activity, resulting in an increase in cardiac output and a higher risk of arrhythmias.

Tracheostomy

Indications

- Upper airway obstruction.
- To facilitate weaning for mechanical ventilation.
- Pulmonary toilet.
- Major head and neck surgery.
- Long-term airway support (neurological disorder or injury).

Tracheostomies are commonly used in ICUs if prolonged mechanical ventilation or weaning difficulties are anticipated. Currently there is no consensus as to when is the optimal time to perform a tracheostomy in these patients. Evidence has generally not demonstrated any mortality benefit in early tracheostomy insertion (≤4 days) versus late (≥10 days). Therefore, the decision to tracheostomise a mechanically ventilated patient is made on an individual case-by-case basis depending on multiple factors including pathology, indications, and illness course and trajectory. Tracheostomies have many advantages over endotracheal tubes including patient comfort, reduced sedation requirements, and improved mouthcare as well as potentially the ability to speak and swallow.

Priority

Elective

The majority of tracheostomies are performed as elective procedures in the operating theatre or ICU.

Urgent

Occasionally tracheostomies are performed under local anaesthesia or careful sedation in patients with upper airway obstruction, in whom conventional intubation is thought to be very difficult or impossible.

Emergency

Performing a tracheostomy requires both time and a skilled operator and therefore is not the recommended first-line technique to obtain emergency front of neck access (eFONA) in the life-threatening event of 'can't intubate, can't oxygenate' (CICO). In such a scenario scalpel cricothyroidotomy is the first-line technique.

Procedure

A tracheostomy can be inserted using a percutaneous or surgical technique.

Percutaneous

A percutaneous procedure can be performed at the bedside on the ICU using a needle, guidewire, and dilator method. A cannula is inserted percutaneously between the first and second or second and third tracheal rings under direct visualisation using a bronchoscope via an endotracheal tube. A guidewire is then passed through the cannula and an introducer then dilator railroaded over the wire to create a sufficiently sized opening to insert a tracheostomy tube.

Surgical

A surgical approach involves dissecting down to the trachea, creating a window into the airway, and inserting a tracheostomy tube. This technique is performed by an ENT surgeon in theatre and often requires two anaesthetists, one to manipulate the endotracheal tube and one to maintain anaesthesia.

Anatomy

- The larynx consists of three large unpaired cartilages (epiglottis, thyroid, and cricoid) and six smaller paired cartilages (arytenoids, cuneiforms, and corniculates), see Fig. 41.1.
- The cricothyroid membrane covers the gap between the thyroid and cricoid cartilage.
- The trachea extends from the lower border of the cricoid cartilage to the carina (15 cm in an adult). It has approximately 20 C-shaped cartilaginous rings, which are deficient posteriorly. The trachealis muscle forms the posterior border of the trachea.
- Motor, sensory, and autonomic innervation of the larynx and trachea come from branches of the vagus nerve (superior and recurrent laryngeal nerves) and from branches of the middle cervical ganglion.
- Large vessels (including the aortic arch) and nerves, as well as the vascular thyroid gland, lie in close proximity to the trachea.

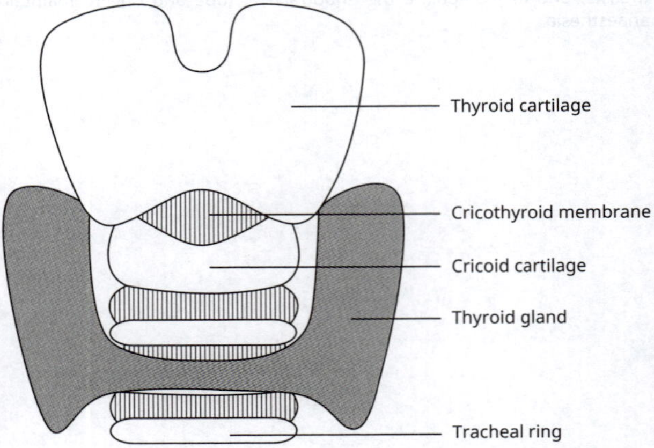

Fig. 41.1 Anatomy

Changes in physiology

- The airway resistance decreases as the upper airway is bypassed.
- Inspired air is not warmed and humidified, as it does not pass through the nose and mouth. This results in increased mucus production and altered colonisation of the upper airways. Therefore, humidification of the inspired gas is essential.
- Cough is severely impaired or impossible, as the patient is unable to produce the high intrathoracic pressures required for coughing, which are usually achieved by straining against a closed glottis.
- The normal swallowing mechanism is impaired because of splinting of the larynx.
- Patients are unable to speak unless the cuff is deflated or special attachments (e.g. speaking valve, fenestrated tube) are used.
- The sense of smell is potentially impaired because of reduced airflow through the nasal passages.

Tracheostomy tubes and attachments

Tracheostomy tubes come in a variety of shapes, lengths, and diameters (Fig.41.2). There are also additional pieces of equipment that can be attached to the tracheostomy.

- ***Fixed or variable length:*** variable (adjustable flange) tubes are used if there is concern that a fixed length tube will not reach the trachea due to increased pre-tracheal space, e.g. obesity and goitre. They are also used if the optimal length of insertion may change over time, for example as a result of swelling in burns patients.
- ***Cuffed or uncuffed:*** uncuffed tubes are used to overcome upper airway obstruction or to facilitate tracheal suctioning of secretions in patients who do not need ventilation and are not at risk of aspiration. Tubes used for ventilation are usually cuffed.
- ***Single or double (with or without an inner tube):*** the inner tube can be removed for cleaning, whilst the outer tube remains in situ.
- ***Fenestrated or non-fenestrated:*** fenestrated tubes have a series of holes in their outer curvature, through which expiratory airflow is directed to pass through the vocal cords to aid phonation. The holes can be blocked off with a non-fenestrated inner tube.
- ***Speaking valves:*** these are one-way valves which are placed on the outer end of the tracheostomy tube. They allow air to be inhaled but close on exhalation, directing the airflow through the vocal cords. Cuffed tubes must be deflated and the upper airway needs to be patent.
- ***Swedish nose:*** is a humidification device that attaches to the tracheostomy to provide passive humidification as the patient breathes.

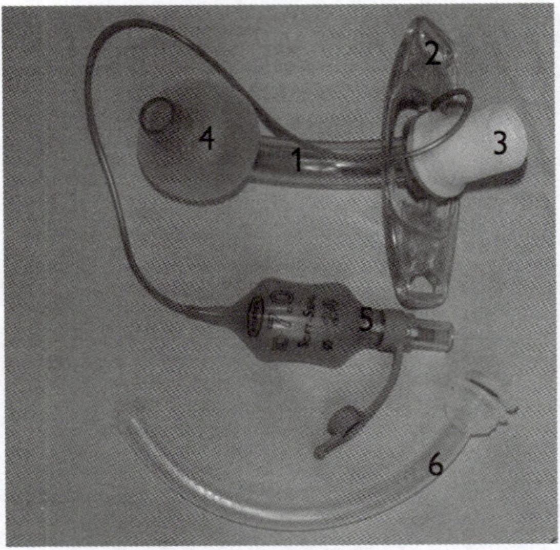

Fig. 41.2 Tracheostomy tubes and attachments: (1) outer cannula; (2) flange/neck plate; (3) 15 mm adaptor; (4) cuff; (5) pilot balloon; (6) inner cannula.

Complications

Immediate (<24 hours)

- Haemorrhage.
- Aspiration.
- Bronchospasm.
- Injury to trachea, larynx, and neighbouring structures.
- Displacement of tube and loss of airway.
- Subcutaneous emphysema, pneumothorax, and pneumomediastinum.
- Procedure failure.

Early (1–14 days)

- Subcutaneous emphysema, pneumothorax, and pneumomediastinum.
- Tube displacement and blockage.
- Wound infection.
- Tracheal necrosis
- Delayed haemorrhage.
- Tracheo-innominate artery fistula (Catastrophic haemorrhage).

Late (>2 weeks)

- Haemorrhage due to erosion into large vessels.
- Tracheal stenosis.
- Tracheomalacia.
- Tracheo-cutaneous or trachea-oesophageal fistula.
- Laryngeal injury.
- Decannulation problems.

General considerations

- ⚠ Call for anaesthetic and ENT help early if there is a tracheostomy emergency.
- ⚠ Changing tracheostomy tubes is associated with considerable risks, particularly in an emergency situation. It should only be performed by appropriately trained and experienced practitioners, who have the knowledge and skills required to manage the airway if the tube exchange fails.
- ⚠ In a recently fashioned tracheostomy (<7 days) a tract has not yet formed, and the stoma may close quickly after the tube has been removed. Percutaneous dilatational stomas may be more prone to collapse than surgical stomas. Early replacement of a tracheostomy tube can be very difficult and carries a high risk of creating a false passage. Positive-pressure ventilation into a false passage can result in rapid development of pneumothorax, pneumomediastinum, and subcutaneous emphysema of neck, larynx, and pharynx. This can render further airway management and ventilation impossible.
- ▶▶Equipment for an emergency tube change should be readily available for each patient with a tracheostomy. This should include:
    - Tracheostomy tubes (same size and one size smaller).
    - Tracheal dilator.
    - Bougie.
    - Stitch cutters.
    - Self-inflatable bag and mask.
    - Oxygen source and tubing.
    - Syringe.
    - Stethoscope.
    - Suction.
- Laryngectomy patients have no connection between their upper airways and their lungs and therefore cannot be oxygenated or ventilated this way.
- The National Tracheostomy Safety Project (NTSP) states that all patients with a tracheostomy must have an airway poster at the end of the bed which includes patient-specific information such as date of insertion, technique for insertion etc., as well as stating if this is a tracheostomy or laryngectomy.
- The poster includes an algorithm for emergency tracheostomy or laryngectomy management.

Tracheostomy emergencies

⚠ Call for anaesthetic and ENT help early.

⚠ Follow NTSP emergency tracheostomy management algorithm.

The most likely tracheostomy emergencies are the loss of the airway due to tube blockage or displacement, bleeding from the tracheostomy, and subcutaneous emphysema.

Tube displacement

This is a medical emergency.

If the tube is visibly displaced but the patient is adequately oxygenating, then the cuff can be deflated, and the tube carefully re-positioned before re-inflating the cuff.

If chest expansion and breath sounds are absent and the tube is patent, then it is not in the trachea and may well be compressing it.

- Deflate the cuff and remove the tube immediately.
- If the patient is breathing spontaneously and there is now good air entry and sufficient airflow across the stoma, administer oxygen via the stoma (not via the face). If this is not possible, cover the stoma with an occlusive dressing and deliver oxygen via a face mask.
- If ventilation is required, cover the stoma and ventilate via the upper airway as in a non-tracheostomy patient and prepare for conventional translaryngeal intubation (see NTSP algorithm, Fig. 41.3).

Obstructed tracheostomy tube

This presents with stridor and difficulty breathing. Assess patency and manage as per NTSP algorithm.

Common causes include;

- *Sputum or blood:* remove and clean the inner tube; suction through the tube with a sterile suction catheter. The tube may need changing.
- *Poor alignment within trachea:* check the head and neck alignment and carefully reposition tube.
- *Herniated cuff:* often helped by carefully deflating the cuff. The tube will need changing.

Subcutaneous emphysema

This can be caused by a poor cuff seal, tube misalignment, or partial tube displacement. It may compromise the airway rapidly.

Tracheostomy bleeding

Early senior review and ENT input is required. Sit patient up. Regular dressing changes. If superficial then manage with compression, surgical clips, and topical anticoagulants (adrenaline or tranexamic acid-soaked gauze).

Manage coagulopathy and blood loss.

>10 ml fresh blood (soaked dressing) is significant and requires immediate review.

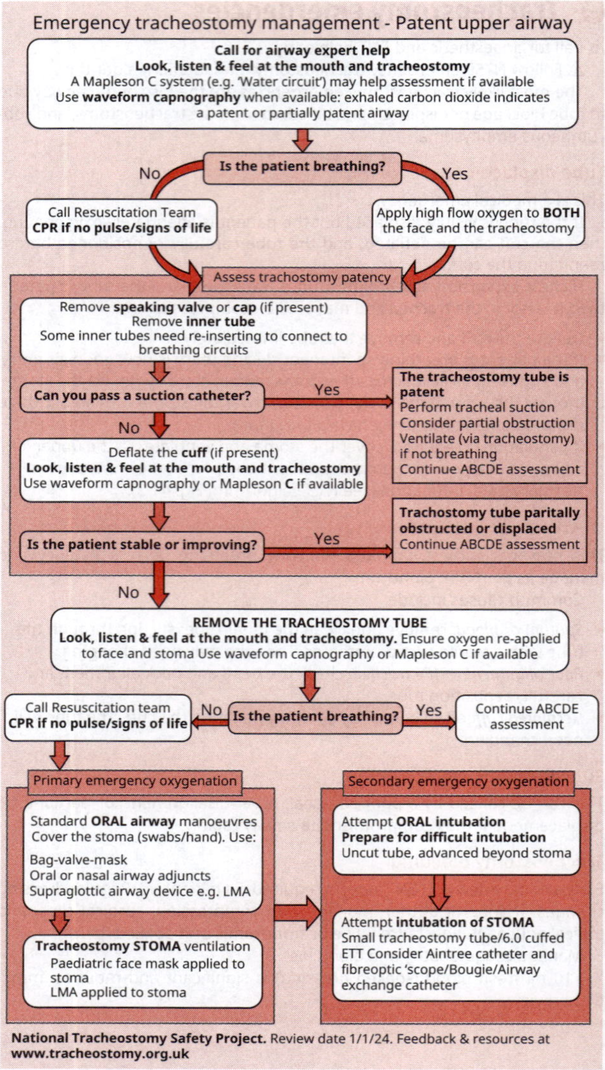

Fig. 41.3 National tracheostomy safety project (NTSP)—Emergency tracheostomy management algorithm. Reproduced with kind permission of the NTSP.

Chapter 42

Oxygen therapy

Introduction

Prompt and correct use of oxygen therapy underpins the management of nearly all respiratory emergencies. Time spent familiarising yourself with local policy and equipment can prove invaluable in the emergency situation.

Principles

The underlying goal of oxygen therapy is to deliver the tissues with an adequate supply to fulfil their metabolic requirement.

Key to this process is the delivery of oxygen (DO_2) equation:

Delivery of oxygen depends on:

(1) Cardiac output, (2) Oxygen content, (3) Haemoglobin

$$DO_2 = \text{cardiac output} \times \text{oxygen content}$$

$$\text{Oxygen content} = \text{Hb} \times SaO_2 \times 1.36 + (PaO_2 \text{ dissolved in plasma} \times 0.023)$$

Oxygen is carried almost entirely by haemoglobin. The amount of oxygen dissolved in plasma contributes <2% which explains why haemoglobin saturation, haemoglobin concentration, and the cardiac output are all important to target in the management of the critically ill patient rather than simply aiming for a PaO_2.

In the emergency setting oxygen therapy should always be considered in the context of the DO_2 and hence as part of a cardiorespiratory resuscitation plan.

Worked example

Critically ill patient with Hb 10 g/dL, PaO_2 8.0 kPa, and SpO_2 92%.

One litre of blood contains:

$$10 \times 0.92 \times 1.36 \times 10(\text{convert litres}) = 125 \text{ml}O_2/\text{L}$$

If the cardiac output is 4 L/min:

$$DO_2 = 4 \times 125 = 500 \text{ml}O_2/\text{min}.$$

↑ FiO_2 to increase SpO_2 to 97%:

$$DO_2 = 10 \times 0.97 \times 1.36 \times 10 = 131.9 \times 4 = 527 \text{ml}O_2/\text{min}.$$

However, if the cardiac output is increased to 5:

$$DO_2 = 125 \times 5 = 625 \text{ml}O_2/\text{min}$$

In this example, increasing the cardiac output has increased oxygen delivery by 25%, whereas just increasing SaO_2 led to a 5% increase.

Combining increases in FiO_2 with adequate resuscitation should enable optimal tissue oxygen delivery.

What is 'controlled' oxygen therapy?

A controlled system is an oxygen delivery system (Table 42.1) that permits the best degree of control over FiO_2. No system is perfect but, for example, a Venturi valve mask allows delivery of a prescribed FiO_2. In contrast, the amount of oxygen delivered by nasal cannulae varies depending upon the respiratory rate and degree of mouth breathing.

Table 42.1 Oxygen delivery systems

Delivery system	Details	FiO_2	Comments
Nasal cannulae	Prong delivered	Not known	Ensure fitted correctly. FiO_2 dependent on flow rate and breathing pattern including respiratory rate and degree of mouth breathing. Not for sole use in emergency. Can be used in combination with other delivery systems.
Venturi mask	Coloured valve system	Flow as advised on valve. FiO_2 is written on valve	System of choice for the hypoxic patient requiring controlled therapy. If remains hypoxic FiO_2 is not increased by increasing flow rate. The valve needs to be changed.
Hudson mask	Simple mask	5–8 L gives 0.5–0.6	Often used as 'default mask' but neither high flow nor controlled.
Reservoir bag	Mask with bag below	10–15 L provides ~0.8	First-line for resuscitation. Start by inflating bag by pressing on valve. Must be fully inflated.
High-flow nasal oxygen	Nasal prong delivered	1.0 with up to 60 L/min flow	Flow flushes out anatomical dead spaces and provides a mild degree of PEEP.
CPAP	Tight-fitting face mask with special delivery system	>0.8 with PEEP	Useful in selected patients with significant hypoxia, e.g. LVF, pneumonia.

In practice: using oxygen in respiratory emergencies

- Supplementation of oxygen in hypoxic critically ill people is given to improve oxygenation. It does not treat underlying pathology causing hypoxia. This must be diagnosed and treated urgently.
- Not all respiratory emergencies require acute oxygen therapy. However, if significant hypoxia is apparent or suspected proceed as below.
- The first priority in an emergency should be to check that the airway and breathing is adequate to 'deliver' oxygen (i.e. ABC).
- Next, commence high-flow oxygen therapy. Use a reservoir bag initially; this provides the maximal FiO_2 at high inspiratory rates; which often exceed the 15 L provided by hospital wall oxygen outlet. Ensure that the reservoir bag is inflated.
- If the patient is known to be oxygen sensitive then deliver oxygen by a controlled system and aim for a saturation that is estimated to be 'normal for the patient' (see below).
- In the emergency setting it is often unclear if a patient is 'sensitive' to oxygen (e.g. COPD in A & E).
- If chronic lung disease is suspected, aim for an oxygen saturation between 88% and 92%.
- Therapy adjustments can be made when further clinical information and ABG results are available.
- Be very careful reducing oxygen in the narcosed hypercarbic patient, e.g. a COPD patient who has been given uncontrolled excess oxygen in ambulance transit and arrives unconscious. Reducing FiO_2 quickly may precipitate cardiac arrest because of the combination of reduced FiO_2 and poor ventilation. Consider short course NIV or, if not available, try respiratory support with Ambubag after discussion with the intensive care team.

Clearly communicate rationale for choice of oxygen delivery system and flow rate to clinical team. Document your strategy and escalation plan in the notes and ensure oxygen is prescribed. In very unwell patients—remember to regularly review the patient and oxygen requirement.

If the patient is oxygen sensitive consider recording this in the hypersensitivity section of the drug chart.

How much oxygen should be given?

- The aim is to provide an adequate supply for tissue oxygenation.
- Normally target saturations for patients is 94–98%, unless they are at risk of hypercapnic respiratory failure—then the target is 88–92%.

Patients with chronic respiratory disorders have often 'adapted' to lower baseline saturations. This may be with or without chronic hypercapnia. Look for clues to help decide if this could be the case:

- History: the underlying diagnosis and severity (FEV_1), use of home oxygen (has a doctor told them to use it for >15 hours/day? Usually LTOT patients have been assessed and should have a PaO2 <7.3 kPa when stable). Previous use of NIV/ventilation.

- Underlying diagnosis that increases risk of chronic hypercapnia are: COPD, morbid obesity, cystic fibrosis, chest wall deformity, neuromuscular disorders. The diagnosis itself does not mean they have chronic hypercapnia—this needs to be assessed on an individual patient basis.
- Examination: respiratory rate may be useful, e.g. if they feel well and RR normal with SaO_2 86%.
- Investigation: perhaps most helpful. Search old notes for previous SaO_2/ABG, especially on discharge or in clinic. Is there evidence of polycythaemia?
- Look at the base excess and bicarbonate: if elevated, suggests compensation for chronic hypercapnia.

If it seems likely that the patient is chronically hypoxic secondary to chronic lung disease, then target oxygen saturations to 88–92% and document in notes. Use clinical response and other markers of tissue oxygenation (e.g. lactate) to ensure adequate therapy.

Oxygen in emergencies: errors to look out for!

- Check tubing from bag/mask is attached to oxygen outlet (not uncommon to find it attached to air outlet in the haste of the moment).
- Acutely hypoxic patient: oxygen flow rate turned up high on venturi mask (valve means effective FiO_2 no greater) or nasal cannulae (not effective).
- 'Non-rebreathe' mask: ensure reservoir bag inflated at onset. Press on valve above bag (the bag provides a sump of oxygen for the high inspiratory flow rate generated).

Chapter 43

Nebulisers

Nebulisers allow the administration of drugs by generating suspensions of particles. They have assumed a central role in the management of patients with acute airways obstruction. However, it should be remembered that most nebulised medication never actually reaches the lung.

Principles and application

- Nebuliser therapy is not an efficient method of administering therapy. Particles are usually either too large or too small to reach the target area (in the acute setting it is estimated that active drug delivery can be as low as 10–20%). Evidence suggests inhalers ± spacing devices are equally, if not more, effective even in the emergency setting.
- In hospital, nebulisers are usually driven by gas or oxygen from the wall outlet supply. In nearly all circumstances use oxygen. To optimise drug delivery it is important that the supply is run at a flow rate of 6 L/minute. If the patient is hypoxic at this flow rate, use nasal cannulae with oxygen simultaneously.
- There is often concern regarding the use of oxygen to drive nebulisers in patients with COPD. It is unlikely that the patient will deteriorate during the course of a supervised nebulised treatment. However, if there is concern and the patient is hypoxic, then use oxygen via nasal cannulae and air to drive the nebuliser (at 6 L/minute).
- Consider changing to inhalers as soon as possible in the hospital admission. Evidence supports the efficacy of inhalers in the acute setting and early prescription allows more time to educate and check inhaler technique.
- Nebulisers for outpatient use should only be prescribed by those with specialist knowledge.

Nebulised therapies

The majority of these therapies are highly specialised. It is always advisable to check local protocol before considering specialised therapies.

- *Antibiotics*. This route of administration has been successfully used in patients with bronchiectasis and cystic fibrosis, e.g. colistimethate sodium, tobramycin, aztreonam, levofloxacin, and gentamicin. Some antibiotics can precipitate acute bronchospasm.
- *Saline*. Saline nebules are thought to free secretions and improve mucus clearance. There is limited evidence of efficacy. In cystic fibrosis patients nebulised 7% saline has been shown to have beneficial effects on lung function. In non-CF bronchiectasis there is evidence that normal saline nebules have a beneficial role as an adjunct to physiotherapy. In a meta-analysis no difference was observed when comparing the use of normal and hypertonic saline nebules, although this is limited by differences in study methodology and patient groups.
- *DNase*. This therapy is widely used as part of the long-term management of CF patients.
- *Antifungals*. Nebulised pentamidine is used in the prophylaxis and treatment of *Pneumocystis jirovecii*, and liposomal amphotericin B is used in the treatment of invasive fungal infections, mainly in the immunocompromised.
- *Tranexamic acid*. In patients with mild haemoptysis nebulised tranexamic acid can be considered. There is some evidence it can reduce bleeding time and reduce the need for further intervention.
- *Iloprost and Treprostinil*. Only for use by PH specialist centres for the treatment of idiopathic or familial pulmonary hypertension (➔ Chapter 35) but has to be given 6–9 times a day.

Chapter 44

Non-invasive ventilation

Non-invasive ventilation

Non-invasive ventilation (NIV) refers to the delivery of ventilatory support via the upper airway using a face or nasal mask. In this chapter NIV refers to non-invasive positive pressure ventilation; negative pressure ventilation (e.g. external cuirass) is not used in the acute setting and will not be discussed. Ventilators can be either pressure or volume controlled, but bi-level pressure support ventilators are by far the most commonly used.

Continuous positive airway pressure (CPAP) is not generally considered to be ventilatory support but is indicated in the acute management of specific clinical scenarios to improve oxygenation.

Bi-level positive airway pressure (BiPAP)

Mechanism of action

The aim of NIV is to decrease the work of breathing, improving alveolar ventilation whilst resting the respiratory muscles. The inspiratory pressure delivered provides increased ventilation to help eliminate carbon dioxide, whilst the expiratory pressure provides improved alveolar ventilation (by preventing the pressure-related collapse of small airways) and recruits under-ventilated lung so improving oxygenation. The difference between the inspiratory and expiratory pressure is the pressure support. High pressure support leads to increased tidal volume, improving ventilation, and removal of carbon dioxide.

Indications

- Patients with an acute exacerbation of COPD in whom a respiratory acidosis (pH <7.35 and pCO_2 >6.5 kpA) persists despite maximal medical treatment on controlled oxygen therapy.
- Acute on chronic hypercapnic ventilatory failure due to chest wall deformity or neuromuscular disease. Consider NIV if pCO_2 >6.5 OR pH <7.35 and pCO_2 >6.5. Patient does not always have to be acidotic for patients with neuromuscular disease to start NIV.
- Obesity hypoventilation—or patients with a history of obstructive sleep apnoea, particularly if acidotic. pH <7.35, pCO_2 >6.5 kpA, or if daytime pCO_2 >6 and somnolent.
- NIV is used in a variety of other settings on the ICU (e.g. acute respiratory distress syndrome, acute pneumonia with hypoxaemia) where tracheal intubation can occur if NIV fails. NIV should not be used for these conditions outside the ICU (unless it has been agreed the patient is not appropriate for ICU transfer).
- NIV should not be used in acute asthma.

Absolute contraindications

- Facial trauma or burns.
- Fixed upper airway obstruction.
- Undrained pneumothorax. Intercostal chest drain should be inserted to treat pneumothorax prior to starting NIV.
- If pneumothorax is too small to be drained—NIV may proceed with careful monitoring. If patient deteriorates then NIV should be discontinued and CXR should be repeated urgently.

Relative contraindications

In some patients NIV is used as the ceiling of treatment, in which case it may be started despite the presence of one or more of the following:

- Vomiting—This is an issue if the NIV mask cannot be removed rapidly, i.e. in patients with neuromuscular weakness or low GCS. An assessment needs to be made about the safety of the patient using NIV and being able to indicate when they want to vomit.
- Haemodynamic instability.
- Confusion or agitation—May make NIV difficult to apply but should not preclude its use.
- Excessive secretions.
- Severe hypoxaemia or acidosis.

- Inability to protect airway. If a patient has NIV as their ceiling of care, a low GCS or GCS <8 does not preclude them from a trial of NIV.
- Advanced age alone should not preclude a trial of NIV

Factors predicting success
These include younger age, lower APACHE scores, and less severe blood gas parameters. Those who are able to cooperate and coordinate better with the machine also have better outcomes.

Setting up non-invasive ventilation

The aim of using NIV is to reduce arterial carbon dioxide levels, improve oxygenation, and correct arterial pH. NIV allows us to buy time to treat the underlying cause of the respiratory failure. Ideally NIV should be started in patients within 60 minutes of blood gas results.

Patients should be on maximal medical therapy and controlled oxygen and fit the criteria as outlined above.

Prior to starting NIV:

- All patients starting on NIV should have an agreed ceiling of care prior to set up. If patients are for full escalation, there should be a plan for escalation if NIV does not work and also a discussion of whether invasive mechanical ventilation is more appropriate for initial treatment.
- Explain to the patient the use of the machine and the mask.
- Select a mask that will fit the patient.
- Set up the ventilator: usual starting pressures are IPAP 10 for patients with COPD, Obesity hypoventilation syndrome, or chest wall disease. Uptitrate the IPAP to 20–30 over 10–30 minutes to achieve adequate ventilation and good chest wall movement. EPAP 4, with a back-up breath rate of 10–15.
- IPAP 10 in patients with neuromuscular disease and EPAP 4, with a back-up breath rate of 10–15.
- Ensure that a bacterial filter is included in circuit.
- Commence NIV holding the mask in place for the first few minutes to allow the patient to become used to it.
- Secure the mask with head straps.
- Monitor pulse oximetry.
- Entrain oxygen if required—the closer to the mask the better. Aim for oxygen saturations of 88–92%. In patients with chest wall disease or neuromuscular disease—you can aim for oxygen saturations of above 92%.
- Monitor respiratory rate, blood pressure, and heart rate.
- Repeat ABGs in 1 hour.
- Use NIV for as much time as possible for the first 24 hours, with breaks for comfort if patient wants.
- NIV use is then gradually reduced and the patient has prolonged periods of self-ventilation slowly over 48–72 hours depending on patients work of breathing and ABG results. This should be done with expert review.

Monitoring

- Conscious level.
- Patient comfort.
- Chest wall motion.
- Accessory muscle use.

- Coordination of respiration with the ventilator.
- Respiratory rate.
- Heart rate.
- Oxygen saturation.
- Repeat ABGs at 1 hour.
- Repeat ABGs at 4 hours if not improving.

Treatment failure

This can occur because of a failure of the gases to improve, an inability for the patient to tolerate NIV, a deterioration in the patient's general condition, or a development of new symptoms.

- Ensure optimal medical treatment of underlying cause – i.e. COPD treatment.
- Confirm that all prescribed treatment is being administered (there should be a break in NIV to deliver nebulisers if they cannot be given simultaneously).
- Consider chest physiotherapy to alleviate sputum retention.
- Exclude any complications such as pneumothorax or aspiration, or complication of associated comorbidity.
- Check that ventilator and circuit are set up correctly.

If ABG not improving after NIV has been set up:

- Check that the patient is not over-oxygenated
- Check the mask is fitting adequately
- Is the patient able to use the machine? If patients are claustrophobic or agitated, they may need reassurance and closer nursing care. Sedatives can be considered to help with compliance.
- Is the patient able to synchronise with the ventilator?

If the above are not an issue or corrected and $PaCO_2$ remains high, consider increasing IPAP.

- If PaO_2 remains low, consider increasing oxygen or increasing EPAP.
- Note—Patients with OHS may require a higher EPAP to help with alveolar recruitment. This will improve oxygenation.
- If patient is for intubation and ventilation—consider need for escalation to critical care for invasive mechanical ventilation.
- Remember to seek help from the on-call Respiratory Team if you need help with the patient and ventilator settings.

Other Uses of bi-level positive airway pressure

Cystic fibrosis/bronchiectasis

NIV is often used successfully for acute exacerbations associated with acidosis and hypercapnia, particularly in end-stage disease where this may be the ceiling of treatment. Its use is sometimes limited by excessive secretions.

Weaning in the intensive care unit

NIV has been used successfully to wean in the ICU setting, with some studies showing reduced intubation time, reduced ICU stay, and reduced incidence of ventilator-associated pneumonia.

Cardiogenic pulmonary oedema

NIV has not been shown to be superior to CPAP.

Continuous positive airway pressure (CPAP)

CPAP is used in those with acute respiratory failure (type 1 respiratory failure) to correct hypoxaemia. It improves oxygenation by increasing mean airway pressure, thus increasing ventilation to collapsed areas of lung, recruiting under-ventilated areas of lung, and thereby correcting ventilation–perfusion mismatch and shunting. It also reduces inspiratory work, decreasing the work of breathing.

Uses of continuous positive airway pressure

Cardiogenic pulmonary oedema

CPAP has been shown to be an effective treatment in pulmonary oedema for patients who remain hypoxic despite maximal medical therapy. A number of randomised controlled studies showed a reduction in intubation rates and a reduced mortality.

Pneumonia

CPAP has been used in the treatment of severe community-acquired pneumonia as well as in the treatment of pneumocystis pneumonia in the immunocompromised, where patients remain hypoxic despite maximal medical therapy. CPAP improves oxygenation, reduces respiratory rate, and reduces dyspnoea.

Ideally, CPAP should be used in an HDU/ICU setting for these patients where intubation would be required in the event of treatment failure with CPAP.

Obstructive sleep apnoea

The most common use for CPAP is in the long-term management of obstructive sleep apnoea, where it acts as an upper airway 'splint' to eliminate apnoeic episodes.

Further reading

BTS/ICS Guideline for the Ventilatory Management of Acute Hypercapnic Respiratory Failure in Adults. 2016. Available online at https://www.brit-thoracic.org.uk/

Chapter 45

Intensive care referral

Intensive care medicine

Intensive care medicine generally involves acutely managing critically unwell patients that require invasive organ support to survive. However, it is not limited to this, with some patients requiring closer monitoring, enhanced nursing care, or optimisation of their ongoing medical management that can only be provided in a critical care environment. A patient's problems and care needs may be relatively straightforward requiring a single intervention such as a patient with an exacerbation of COPD and type II respiratory failure requiring non-invasive ventilation (NIV). Very often, however, patients are complex requiring invasive multi-organ support, e.g. a patient with chest sepsis and subsequent multi-organ dysfunction.

The common respiratory reasons for requesting ICU input are as follows:

- Hypoxemic (Type I) respiratory failure (oxygenation failure), which is either approaching the maximum percentage of oxygen (FiO_2) that can be provided at ward level or is complicated by an altered mental state or additional organ dysfunction.
- Hypercapnic (Type II) respiratory failure (ventilatory failure) without a clear and reversible cause such as an acute exacerbation of COPD or opiate toxicity is likely to require some form of ventilatory support.
- Upper airway emergencies.
- Non respiratory organ failure secondary to underlying respiratory pathology, e.g. circulatory or renal support because of severe chest sepsis.

It is not possible to be prescriptive about whom to admit to the ICU and when to admit them. Each patient must be assessed and managed on a case-by-case basis with consideration of multiple factors including underlying pathology, trajectory of illness, and response to treatment, comorbidities, physical reserve, functional capacity, prognosis, and patient wishes. However, certain principles apply and, if followed, will make for fruitful discussion with intensive care doctors and effective patient care.

Involve ICU early

Many patients admitted to ICU, or suffering a cardiac arrest in hospital, show physiological signs of deterioration for hours and days prior to this event. Hospital early warning scoring systems have been developed and validated to help identify sick and deteriorating patients that may require an escalation of their care. Involvement of the critical care team is one such escalation and this should be considered early in appropriate patients that appear to be deteriorating despite ward level care. Early ICU awareness and review may not only optimise the patient's current medical management but also allows the parent and ICU team to plan for different eventualities together and facilitates patient and family discussions regarding treatment options and ceilings of care.

Ensure early resuscitation and maximum therapy

Early resuscitation of the unwell patient is essential with implications for both short- and long-term outcomes. This is best demonstrated in the Surviving Sepsis guidelines that recommend early intravenous fluid resuscitation and antimicrobial administration in patients with sepsis. Before referring to ICU, ensure that all possible care has been initiated on the ward or in the ED.

What can ICU offer?

Remember that intensive care cannot fix all pathologies. It can provide organ support, close monitoring, and enhanced nursing care whilst the patient hopefully responds to medical or surgical therapy. If the patient is unlikely to respond to therapy and recover from the acute illness, then intensive care admission is unlikely to change this and will merely prolong suffering and death. ICU interventions have significant risks attached to them and deleterious consequences. Indeed, much of the benefit of NIV in COPD is in avoiding endotracheal intubation with its subsequent risks of ventilator-associated pneumonia.

Consider comorbidities

The best that any patient can hope for is to return to their premorbid level of function. Patients with multiple comorbidities, pre-existing organ dysfunction, reduced physical reserve, and poor functional status are very unlikely to return to anything like their baseline and are much more likely to have a poor outcome to their ICU stay.

COPD

COPD patients requiring NIV should have a clear plan regarding ceilings of care. There is often a nihilistic approach to invasive ventilation for COPD, although published data from the Intensive Care National Audit and Research Centre (ICNARC) suggest that patients with single organ failure, good functional status, lack of other organ dysfunction (including poor nutritional status), and a reversible disease process have a survival to discharge of 70%. This is comparable with many conditions for which admission to ICU is not debated. Age and FEV_1 should not be used in isolation when assessing suitability. Functional status, BMI, oxygen requirements when stable, comorbidities, and previous admissions to the ICU should also be considered.

Convalescence

A medical patient admitted to the ICU is likely to have a prolonged hospital admission, including tracheostomy to facilitate weaning from ventilatory support. Following discharge from the ICU patients often require high levels of ongoing care with both physical and psychological rehabilitation. Return to premorbid function may not occur, and even in those in whom it does, it can take many months and even years.

Discussion with patient and relatives

In an ideal situation and time permitting discussions with patients and their families should take place prior to ICU involvement. In some scenarios, admission to the ICU for invasive organ support is the patient's best, and sometimes only, chance of survival and a positive outcome. Many patients and families knowing that will want to do all they can despite the risks involved. However, this may require a prolonged ICU and hospital stay, invasive procedures and multiple medications and therapies that all carry risks of complications such as acquired infections and delirium with no guarantee of a return to an acceptable quality of life at the end of it all.

For many patients the reality of ICU is not something they would wish or accept and, in that case, alternative options such as conservative medical management or palliative care may be best for them. These discussions may be outside the experience or competency of the ward doctor. If needed, the ICU team should be involved to discuss these issues with the family even if ICU care is not a realistic option.

Mechanical ventilation

This refers to ventilation via an endotracheal tube or tracheostomy to enable the delivery of high inspired fractions of oxygen, effective PEEP, and control of tidal volume and respiratory rate to improve the clearance of CO_2.

There are many ventilatory modes available which all have subtle difference however they broadly fit into one of two categories.

- Pressure control ventilation (PCV): tidal volume is determined by preset pressures and respiratory system compliance.
- Volume control ventilation (VCV): a preset tidal volume is delivered, and the airway pressures are then a consequence of the respiratory mechanics.

The use of lung protective ventilation with low tidal volumes, limiting plateau pressures, and consequent permissive hypercapnia has been shown to reduce ventilator-induced lung injury and improve survival in ARDS. Lung protective ventilation has now been adopted across the board and used for most ICU patients requiring ventilatory support.

Some patients in ICU are totally dependent on mechanical ventilation, performing only mandated breaths from the ventilator and not putting in any intrinsic breaths of their own. This may be to do directly with their underlying pathology or severity of disease or may be a deliberate action through sedative and/or paralytics agents to strictly control ventilation and gas exchange in certain clinical scenarios such as traumatic brain injury.

Other ICU patients require only 'partial' ventilatory support and do some or most of the work of breathing themselves depending on their ventilatory mode and setting. They will trigger the ventilator themselves at a time determined by their own respiratory drive and then receive a level of pressure support to help produce an effective tidal volume and overcome the work of breathing of the airway. This helps to reduce muscle wasting and aids with the weaning process.

Chapter 46

Pre-operative assessment

Introduction

A pre-operative assessment is an essential tool to determine a patient's peri-operative risk.

The pre-operative assessment includes:

- Thorough history including a review of patient risk factors.
- Physical examination including airway assessment.
- Review of previous anaesthetic charts and relevant clinic letters.
- Collate investigation findings.
- Referral for specialist medical input if required, e.g. cardiology and respiratory.

The information acquired enables the medical and surgical teams to quantify the patient's peri-operative risks and aids in their decision-making process to ensure the best for the patient.

- Investigations, specialist team referrals, and subsequent medication and lifestyle changes can be made pre-operatively to optimise the patient's cardio-respiratory function prior to surgery.
- Decisions can be made early as to the most appropriate anaesthetic and surgery to provide for a patient given their comorbidities and functional state.
- The level of post-operative care and support the patient is likely to require can be determined and arrangements can be made.

The findings of the pre-operative assessment and its implications can then be discussed with the patient and their family. This affords the patient the best opportunity to weigh up the information given, to come to a decision that is best for them, and provide us with informed consent.

Peri-operative respiratory function

There are many factors that increase the risk of a patient developing respiratory complications during the peri-operative period.

Patient factors

- Pre-existing respiratory disease (COPD, OSA)
- Other significant comorbidities, especially cardiovascular disease.
- Poor performance and functional capacity.
- Smoking.
- Obesity.
- Increased age.

Surgical factors

- Upper abdominal and thoracic surgery (reluctance to cough, development of atelectasis and sputum retention).
- Prolonged surgery (>3.5 hours).

Anaesthetic factors

- General anaesthesia leads to several changes in respiratory physiology.
- Relaxation of muscles → atelectasis in dependent areas.
- Reduced functional residual capacity (FRC) → Prone to hypoxaemia.
- Increased closing volume encroaching on FRC → Prone to hypoxaemia.
- Decreased response to hypoxaemia, hypercarbia, and acidosis.

History

A thorough history is required to ascertain the patient's current health, their comorbidities, and their functional performance. Patients should be specifically asked about the following:

- Current symptoms—Cough, sputum, dyspnoea.
- Extent of dyspnoea.
- Ability to lie flat.
- Recent infection, worsening symptoms, or decline in exercise tolerance.
- Cigarette consumption.
- Subjective assessment of functional capacity—How far can you walk? Can you climb stairs? Can you perform all ADLs?
- Respiratory comorbidities (COPD, OSA).
- Other comorbidities that may affect respiratory system (e.g. cardiac).
- Type of treatment and usual response (optimally controlled?).
- Previous hospital admissions, operations, ICU admissions.

Examination

Look for abnormal findings, especially for complications of respiratory disease, such as pulmonary hypertension, right heart failure, steroid effects, and cachexia.

Functional

Simply asking the patient to lie flat and to climb stairs can provide very useful information.

Investigations

Depending on the information acquired from the history and examination, investigations may be indicated to formally assess the patients cardio-respiratory function and objectively determine their functional capacity.

CXR

Request if history or clinical signs are suggestive of chest or cardiac disease.

ECG

Request for every patient >60 years and for younger patients if cardiovascular or significant respiratory disease are present or suspected.

Spirometry

May provide useful information in the following circumstances.

- Evidence of significant respiratory disease.
- Equivocal clinical findings and uncertainty of diagnosis.
- Inability to ascertain exercise tolerance in patients with lower limb disability.
- To assess reversibility of pulmonary obstruction with beta-agonists or steroids.
- Prior to parenchymal lung resection.

FEV_1 <1 L increases the likelihood of post-operative respiratory complications and need for post-operative ventilation.

6-minute walk test (6MWT)

This measures how far a patient can walk on the flat in 6 minutes. Measurements include oxygen saturations, heart rate, 6-min walk distance (6MWD), modified Borg dyspnoea scale, and leg fatigue.

Cardiopulmonary exercise testing (CPET)

This is a non-invasive objective method of evaluating both cardiac and pulmonary function. It may help to differentiate between cardiac and respiratory causes of dyspnoea. Variables measured include maximum oxygen consumption and anaerobic threshold.

Arterial blood gases

ABGs can identify chronic hypercapnic respiratory failure and are useful as a pre-operative baseline test in those with chronic respiratory disease. An elevated $PaCO_2$ increases peri-operative risk.

Echocardiogram (ECHO)

Useful to assess ventricular function and rule out valvular disease in patients with unexplained dyspnoea and those with clinical and/or ECG evidence of cardiac disease.

Cigarette smoking

Effects

- Associated with COPD, cardiovascular disease, and lung malignancy.
- Reduced mucociliary clearance.
- Increased airway reactivity → increased risk of coughing, bronchospasm, and laryngospasm.
- Increased COHb → reduced oxygen delivery (5–15% COHb in heavy smokers).
- Nicotine stimulates the sympathetic system → increasing cardiac workload and coronary vascular resistance.

Cessation

- It takes at least 8 weeks abstinence to see major benefits and reduced morbidity. In fact, cessation of <8 weeks may increase airway reactivity.
- Patients who are unable to stop smoking >8 weeks prior to surgery may still benefit from a 12–24 hour cessation, during which the nicotine and COHb levels normalise.

Obstructive sleep apnoea (OSA)

The STOP-BANG screening tool for OSA is a useful aid to identify potentially undiagnosed OSA patients during the pre-operative assessment.

In patients who are intermediate or high risk, then consider referral for overnight pulse-oximetry or sleep study if surgery can be delayed. In more urgent patients then consider pre-operative continuous positive airway pressure (CPAP).

Other pre-operative management options

- Optimise medical management of pre-existing respiratory disease, e.g. inhalers, nebulisers, and steroids.
- A pre-operative course of antibiotics if there is evidence of infection.
- Referral for pulmonary rehabilitation prior to surgery.
- Chest physiotherapy input.
- Weight loss if obese.
- Dietician referral to optimise nutrition if underweight or malnourished.

Resources

Silvapulle, E and Darvall, J. Subjective methods for preoperative assessment of functional capacity. BJA Education 2022; 22 (7): 249–257.

Silvapulle, E and Darvall, J. Objective methods for preoperative assessment of functional capacity. BJA Education 2022; 22 (8): 312–320.

Chapman, S.J., Robinson, G.V., Shrimanker, R., Turnbull, C.D. and Wrightson, J.M. (2021). *Oxford Handbook of Respiratory Medicine 4e*. Oxford: Oxford University Press USA–OSO.

Chapter 47

Respiratory physiotherapy

Respiratory physiotherapy (PT) is indicated in specific situations. In acute situations it tends to be to facilitate secretion clearance and improve ventilation. PT may also be involved with management of non-invasive ventilation, tracheostomies, weaning, and rehabilitation. A respiratory physiotherapist referral should be considered in the management of certain chronic conditions including breathing pattern disorder, asthma, COPD, bronchiectasis, and cystic fibrosis

Airway clearance techniques

Several airway clearance techniques (ACTs) are available and can be used alone or in combination according to the clinical situation.

- ACBT: the active cycle of breathing techniques is a group of breathing exercises used to aid/facilitate sputum expectoration. The three components are breathing control (BC), thoracic expansion exercises (TEE), and the forced expiration technique (FET).
- Manual techniques (MT) are percussion, vibration, and shakes performed manually by the PT on the patient.
- Autogenic drainage (AD): an airway clearance technique characterised by breathing control, with the emphasis on slow inspiration, then inspiratory pause followed by high expiratory flows whilst avoiding airway closure/collapse. The individual utilizes breathing at VT, varying the depth within the inspiratory/expiratory reserve volumes according to the location of secretions, with the aim of mobilising the secretions centrally from the peripheral airways. AD can be carried out independently or with assistance to apply overpressure.
- Postural drainage (PD) utilises the anatomy of the main airways of the lung to allow specific positioning to drain a specific lung segment. Head down techniques are less commonly used.
- Positive expiratory pressure (PEP) which may including oscillating PEP (OPEP). There are a variety of devices available in the UK (including Pari PEP, Astra PEP, flutter, cornet, Accapella Aerobika). The individual breathes in (no resistance) through the equipment using slightly larger than normal tidal volumes, and then exhales through the device creating a resistance plus/minus oscillation depending on the device. generating a PEP of approximately 10–20 cmH_2O. Most devices allow the resistance to be adjusted. This is repeated five to ten times before performing a FET.
- Intermittent positive pressure breathing (IPPB), also known as the Bird (but can be delivered via other devices). IPPB is an adjunct to other ACTs. It is the application of patient-triggered inspiratory pressure and can be delivered via a mouthpiece, full face mask, or tracheostomy attachment. It is used in facilitating sputum clearance and can in the short-term reduce the work of breathing. It is normally delivered with a respiratory physiotherapist present.
- Assisted cough techniques: these are manual techniques carried out by a trained physiotherapist to augment cough strength during the coughing part of an appropriate airway clearance technique, when it is affected by neuromuscular weakness or mechanical disadvantage.

- CoughAssist (cough insufflation/exsufflation) applies positive and negative pressure to augment cough strength. It is applied via a full- face mask, mouthpiece, or tracheostomy interface.
- Intermittent mandatory percussive ventilation (IMPV)/Percusionnaire: varying frequency, pressure, and inspiratory-to-expiratory ratio to maximise airway clearance.
- Suction: negative pressure via catheter inserted into lower airway via nasopharyngeal route, Guedel airway, tracheostomy, or mini tracheostomy.
- Manual hyperinflation (MHI): can be used in patients with a tracheostomy or ETT who are unable to undertake conventional breathing exercises because of an acute deterioration or level of consciousness. Using the 'bag', the physiotherapist can deliver normal VT, MHI, inspiratory pauses, and fast expiratory releases to mimic huff/cough.
- Appropriate exercise and early mobilisation: this can facilitate sputum clearance and improve lung volume recruitment.

Indications for respiratory physiotherapy

Sputum retention

Sputum retention caused by bronchospasm should be managed medically, followed by physiotherapy if still appropriate. Patients with coexisting pain should have sufficient analgesia to allow full inspiration and cough. 'Wound support' or the use of a cough lock may be of assistance in some cases.

Table 47.1 Interventions for sputum retention

	Pathophysiology	Possible PT intervention
Increased secretions or decreased mucociliary clearance	Increased sputum production, decreased mucociliary clearance, or altered rheological properties of sputum (such as in dehydration, poorly controlled diabetes, or CF)	ACBT, AD, PEP or oscillating PEP devices (i.e. ACTs), manual techniques, exercise, postural drainage, IPPB
Ineffective cough, e.g. neuromuscular disease, decreased conscious level	Inspiratory volume limitation	ACTs, IPPB, NIV, IMPV, CoughAssist, suction (be clear whether for upper or lower airway secretion management)
	Limitation in expiratory force generation	ACTs, assisted cough techniques, CoughAssist, suction, cough lock

Tracheostomy patients

Consider tube patency, suction catheter size, humidification, and nursing lead suction. Ensure patient is referred to specialist tracheostomy MDT team if available. Physiotherapist will be involved to avoid secretion retention. A mix of ACTs, MHI, CoughAssist, IPPB, suction, and early mobilisation can be used.

Volume loss

Table 47.2 Interventions for volume loss

Pathophysiology	Possible PT intervention
Treatment strategies for decreased tidal volume (V_T) due to e.g. pain, fatigue, ↑ work of breathing (WOB), dynamic pulmonary hyperinflation	Consider mobilisation, pain management, TEE, IPPB, MHI, relaxation, breathing control
Localised volume loss, e.g. consolidation, collapse	ACTs, mobilisation, positioning
Respiratory muscle weakness/fatigue	IPPB, NIV (Type II RF), positioning

Other causes of breathlessness

For conditions not amenable to physiotherapy treatment, the PT can advise regarding appropriate oxygen delivery, flow rates, humidification, and high-flow devices.

Positioning can be used to ease breathlessness by managing active versus passive fixing and positions of ease, so that the work of breathing is reduced. V/Q matching can be utilised to optimise gas exchange, therefore easing breathlessness.

Contraindications and precautions

Contraindications to PT interventions should be discussed with the physiotherapist with respect to the individual patient. PT is not appropriate for breathlessness solely caused by the following.

- Pleural effusion/empyema.
- PE.
- Pneumonia (consolidated phase).
- Mass.
- Undrained pneumothorax/haemopneumothorax.
- Pulmonary oedema.
- Bronchospasm.
- Stridor.

On-call physiotherapy services

On-call physiotherapy services vary depending on local hospital policy, which will dictate whether the PT is on site or at home, with a specific time in which to attend a call-out.

The PT will ask specific questions to identify whether the problem is amenable to PT intervention and to identify specific contraindications to possible treatment.

Commonly asked questions

- Main symptom?
- What is the underlying pathology?
- Results of ABGs?
- FiO_2: delivery device, flow rate, humidification, and SaO_2.
- Results of recent CXR specifically regarding acute pathology and contraindications to the use of positive pressure if this is felt to be a possibility, e.g. bullous emphysema, undrained pneumothorax, some forms of lung cancer.
- CVS stability is important with regard to contraindications to some PT techniques.
- Fluid balance: hydration is an important component to sputum clearance.
- Pain management if appropriate: rib fractures, ICD, wound management. A patient may be pain free at rest but may be unable to take a deep breath and/or cough.
- Is the patient able to follow commands?

Further reading

Harden, B. (2003). *An On-call Survival Guide: Emergency Physiotherapy*, pp. 79–118. Churchill Livingstone, Edinburgh. DOI: /10.1016/C2009-0-53588-X

Webber, B.A. *et al.* (1998). Physiotherapy techniques. In Webber BA, Pryor JA, eds. *Physiotherapy for Respiratory and Cardiac Problems*, pp. 137–209. Churchill Livingstone, Edinburgh.

Hough, A. (1997). *Physiotherapy in Respiratory Care: A Problem-Solving Approach to Respiratory and Cardiac Management*. Stanley Thornes, Cheltenham.

Chapter 48

Pleural aspiration

Introduction

Pleural aspiration (thoracocentesis/thoracentesis) for diagnostic and therapeutic purposes is a commonly required procedure. Adequate attention must be paid to sterility and technique to prevent potential complications (bleeding, introduction of infection, and damage to the lung resulting in pneumothorax).

Aspiration may be required for two main medical causes. Firstly, for spontaneous pneumothorax of any size or for a small secondary pneumothorax. Secondly, for pleural effusions, this can be for diagnostic evaluation, to relieve symptoms of breathlessness, to evaluate if the underlying lung is non-expandable, and to guide further pleural procedures.

Complications and relative contraindications

Complications

Pleural aspiration is generally considered to be a low-risk intervention. However, serious complications can lead to significant morbidity, mortality, and healthcare costs, therefore they need to be considered and accounted for.

Potential complications need to be discussed in the consent process, these include:

- Pneumothorax: the most common complication. Procedures at higher risk for iatrogenic pneumothorax are those when larger volumes of fluid are removed, in underweight patients, and are likely related to operator experience and smaller depth of fluid marking.
- Bleeding: uncommon complication but iatrogenic intrapleural haemorrhage can be potentially life-threatening. To reduce this risk, the aspiration site should always be directly above a rib to avoid the neurovascular bundle and a posterior approach should be avoided.
- Re-expansion pulmonary oedema (RPO): rare complication (<1%) but potentially life-threatening, characterised by hypoxaemia and new diffuse alveolar infiltrates which is due to a rapid lung re-expansion. Usually occurs within the first hour after therapeutic aspiration.
- Minor complications include iatrogenic infection, chest discomfort, and failure to conclude a diagnosis from the samples taken.

Relative contraindications

In some circumstances the risk of complications/adverse outcomes is greater; for these patient's caution is required when deciding if it is appropriate to undertake a pleural aspiration.

General

- Uncooperative patient.
- Concurrent use of anticoagulation treatment.
- Coagulopathy.
- Local infection at proposed site of aspiration.

Pneumothorax

- Patients on mechanical ventilation; chest drain is preferred due to risk of tension pneumothorax and bronchopleural fistula formation.
- No safe site for aspiration such as small-volume pneumothorax, lung tethering.

Pleural effusions

- Bedside real-time ultrasound not available to identify procedure site.
- No safe site for aspiration identified on thoracic ultrasound such as very small or posterior fluid collections.

General considerations for pleural aspiration procedures

Operator training and competence

The operator for any pleural procedure should have been adequately trained and it is recommended that all operators monitor procedure outcomes and complication rates.

Procedures need to be clearly documented in medical notes; many Trusts use Local Safety Standards for Invasive Procedures (LocSSIPs).

Consent and pre-procedure written information

Informed consent should be obtained (in written form for pleural procedures) and it is advised that written information is given to the patient prior to the procedure if possible.

Timing of procedures

It is strongly recommended that pleural procedures are undertaken in normal working hours if possible (with the exceptions of emergency cases).

Medication review

There is no clear evidence about bleeding risk associated with pleural procedures in patients who are taking antiplatelet, anticoagulation, or have a coagulopathy. Each case needs to be considered on a patient basis as risk and benefit of interrupting medications and/or need for bridging therapies will differ. For emergency procedures it may not be possible to fully treat factors associated with increased bleeding risk; input from haematology specialist team may be needed.

For elective procedures BTS recommend:

- Warfarin is stopped 5 days prior to procedure with INR checked prior to procedure, confirming INR is ≤1.5.
- Direct oral anticoagulation medication (DOAC) should be stopped 24–48hrs prior to procedure and resumed 1 day after a low-risk procedure and 2–3 days after a high-risk procedure.
- Patients may need to be covered with daily prophylactic heparin if they are high risk for venous thromboembolism.
- Clopidogrel and prasugrel should be stopped for 5 days pre-procedure and ticagrelor for 7 days pre-procedure.
- No clear guidance for phosphodiesterase inhibitors (dipyridamole) but most local recommendations would advise holding for 24 hours pre-procedure.
- Aspirin and prophylactic LMWH can be continued.

Environment

It is advised that all pleural procedures should be undertaken in a clean, dedicated pleural procedure room; bedside procedures should be avoided.

Pre-procedural investigations

Full blood count, urea, and electrolytes and liver function tests are usually conducted prior to procedure. Coagulation profile is generally not required if there is no history of coagulopathy, clinical reason to suspect coagulopathy, or use of anticoagulants.

Pre-procedural imaging

A recent CXR or CT scan should be available to review indication and site of pathology.

Thoracic ultrasound must be used at the bedside in real time prior to every procedure with the marking of the most appropriate site intervention. This should be undertaken in the position the procedure is done.

Ultrasound is generally not required in patients with a pneumothorax but may be helpful if there is tethered lung or in cases of loculated pneumothorax.

Local anaesthetic

Lidocaine 1% is the most commonly used local anaesthetic. There is no consensus on maximal dose, but BTS note that up to a dose of 4–5 mg/kg (max. 300 mg=30 ml) have been used without significant increase in side effects.

Larger volumes (rather than dose) of local anaesthetic appear to improve efficacy therefore 1% lidocaine is recommended over 2% preparation.

Post-procedure imaging

A CXR should be performed post-procedure if the patient develops symptoms which do not resolve quickly after the aspiration if the procedure was complicated or if there were multiple aspiration attempts.

Pleural fluid investigations

Advised tests for all sampled pleural effusions:

- Biochemistry (LDH and protein): send 2–5 ml in plain container or in serum blood collection tube depending on local policy. Send serum biochemistry as paired samples. Use Light's criteria to assess if fluid is exudative.
- Microscopy and culture and sensitivity (MC&S): send 5 ml in plain container. If infection is suspected send further 5 ml in both aerobic and anaerobic blood culture bottles.
- Cytology and cell count: Send at least 25 ml in plain universal container.
- Glucose: 1–2 ml in fluoride oxidate tube to be sent to biochemistry.

Other tests to send in selected cases:

- pH: 0.5–1 ml in ABG heparinised blood gas syringe. In non-purulent effusions when pleural infection is suspected.
- Acid-fact bacilli and TB culture: request with MC&S sample.
- Triglycerides and cholesterol: send further sample 2–5 ml if milky effusion aspirated to distinguish chylothorax from pseudochylothorax.
- Amylase: request with biochemistry to assess for pancreatitis-related effusion.
- Haematocrit: 1–2 ml sent in a EDTA container, >50% of serum HCT supports diagnosis of haemothorax.
- Flow cytometry and cytogenetics: send further sample to haematological lab if concerns about haematological malignancy.
- Pleural fluid ADA: in areas of high TB prevalence can be a rule out test for TB pleuritis.

Diagnostic aspiration

- Obtain written consent from the patient.
- Review a recent CXR or CT scan to confirm side of the chest with effusion.
- The patient needs to be positioned comfortably in a stable position with adequate access to chosen aspiration site for the operator.
- Possible positions include patient sitting upright and leaning forward with their arms raised and resting on a table in front of them or lying flat on their side in the fetal position to allow easy access to the safety triangle.
- Aspiration site.
  - Use point of care thoracic ultrasound (TUS) in real time to assess effusion and mark most appropriate site for aspiration.
  - Approach may be posterior or lateral (mid-axillary line).
  - Avoid most posterior area (within about 3 cm of the erector spinae) as the intercostal artery often lies in the mid-intercostal space here.
- Prepare the skin (alcohol-based skin preparation) + aseptic technique.
- Infiltrate local anaesthetic.
  - Use 1% lidocaine 5–10 ml.
  - Initially raise a subcutaneous 'bleb'.
  - Advance while aspirating, aiming for just above the rib (avoids inferiorly placed neurovascular bundle).
  - Infiltrate tissues from skin through intercostal muscle to parietal pleura (may be painful).
  - You may feel a 'give' as you enter the pleural space.
- Aspirate fluid along anaesthetised tract (50 ml syringe, 21G needle/ green).
- Dress insertion area with a sterile dressing.
- Note pleural fluid appearance.
- Send samples of fluid investigations as previously discussed.
- Post-procedure CXR is not routinely required.

Therapeutic aspiration

The same technique as for diagnostic aspiration is used (first six steps above) initially. Then proceed as follows:

- Use of large-bore thoracentesis needle-catheter devices are generally used now for therapeutic aspiration. These are flexible catheters (often 6Fg) which are designed specifically for therapeutic aspirations,
- These needle-catheter devices are usually attached to the draining tubing with a three-way tap and a 30–50 ml syringe.
- This device is inserted along the anaesthetised tract (above the rib). You may feel a 'give' as you enter the pleural space as the parietal pleura is penetrated.
- When fluid or blood can be easily aspirated insert the catheter to hilt into the pleural space and withdraw the needle. The catheter will be left within the chest.
- Fluid can now be aspirated; this is often via gravity drainage into a collection bag or via manual syringe aspiration using a 50 ml syringe (expelled via the three-way tap into a jug).
- Continue aspirating until resistance on aspiration OR significant cough/ chest discomfort/shortness of breath OR 1.5 L has been aspirated (possibly avoids risk of re-expansion pulmonary oedema). Slower, more controlled drainage is thought to reduce the risk of RPO but allows lung to re-expand more gradually.
- Note: removal of as little as 500 ml of fluid may result in substantial therapeutic benefit even in massive pleural effusion (as this decompresses hemithorax and improves respiratory mechanics).
- Dress insertion area with a sterile dressing.
- Repeat CXR after procedure (demonstrates degree of improvement or presence of pneumothorax).

Pneumothorax aspiration

The same technique (sterile preparation, skin infiltration) as above is used, with the following important differences.

- The patient is positioned lying at 45 degrees.
- The approach is anterior: second intercostal space in the mid-clavicular line.
- Pneumothorax is confirmed on aspirating air freely with the 21G local anaesthetic needle.
- Insert a cannula and along the anesthetised tract at a 90-degree angle.
- Begin to remove the needle once at the depth air was aspirated but advance the plastic sheath to the hilt. Attach a three-way tap to the cannula and a 50 ml syringe to the three-way tap.
- Air is expelled via the three-way tap.
- Continue aspirating until resistance on aspiration OR significant cough or chest discomfort OR >2.5 L air aspirated (implies large air leak)—intercostal drainage is likely to be needed.
- Dress insertion area with a sterile dressing.
- Repeat CXR to document 'successful' aspiration.

Chapter 49

Chest drain insertion

Introduction

Although chest drains are used frequently, it should be remembered that there is a significant morbidity and even mortality associated with chest drain insertion.

Complications increase with inexperienced operators, and the procedure must be undertaken or supervised by clinicians with experience in drain insertion. Chest drains are sometimes unnecessarily inserted and careful thought should be given to the indication in each case and potential alternative management strategies.

Intercostal chest drains

The size of an intercostal chest drain is measured in 'French' units. These come in small-bore which is usually ≤14F and large-bore for larger sizes. French units describe the outer diameter and are equal to one third of a mm of their French unit value, thus 12F drain has an outer diameter of 4 mm.

The operator needs to consider indication, their training, and expertise when deciding on what type of chest drain to insert in each patient. Small-bore drains are likely to cause less pain for the patient but have more tendency to kink or block. The majority of drains inserted in the UK are Seldinger drains.

Trocar drain

- Stiff metal rod with a blunt end (trocar) sheathed in a plastic chest drain.
- Normally large size (particularly >20F).
- Inserted using blunt dissection technique (see below).
- Attempted insertion by exerting excessive pressure through the trocar on the chest wall can result in penetrating injury to the lung, heart, and great vessels, and may result in death.

Portex drain

- Similar plastic drain to above, but trocar is replaced with a flexible plastic introducer.
- Inserted using blunt dissection technique.

Seldinger drain

- Smaller flexible drains inserted using the Seldinger technique (guidewire).
- Usually available between 6–18F in commercial kits.
- See section on insertion technique for further details.
- Although insertion technique is perceived to be 'easier' than for trocar or Portex drains, experience is required to prevent complications.

Radiologically inserted drain

- Generally smaller (<14F); inserted by Seldinger technique.
- Can be inserted using ultrasound or CT.
- Consider requesting image guidance if in doubt concerning radiological appearance.
- Particularly useful in multiloculated collections (especially empyema).

Indications for drain insertion

There are no absolute contraindications for insertion of a chest drain especially in an emergency; relative contraindications are similar to those for pleural aspiration discussed in ➲ Chapter 48.

- Tension pneumothorax.
- Pneumothorax not responding to other treatments.
- Symptomatic pleural effusions in patients on mechanical ventilation.
- Simple drainage of large benign or malignant pleural effusions.
- Talc pleurodesis.
- Pleural infection.
- Traumatic haemothorax and/or pneumothorax.
- Post-thoracic cavity procedure such as medical thoracoscopy thoracic/oesophageal/cardiac surgery.

Which size of drain to use?

Seldinger chest drains up to 12F are adequate for most situations. Larger drains are advocated for treatment in patients with a substantial air leak (in trauma, secondary pneumothorax, or ventilated patients), post-cardiac surgery, and acute traumatic haemothorax. In these situations 28–32F drains would be adequate.

There are no adequately powered clinical trials to guide optimal chest drain size selection. Observational studies suggest that smaller drains may be as effective and less painful than larger drains. It is recommended that 18F chest drains may be the optimal size for drains inserted for talc pleurodesis.

Complications of chest drain insertion

Chest drain insertion is generally a safe procedure, however it is associated with an 8–20% complication rate. Complications include:

- Pain.
- Infection (empyema results in up to 1%).
- Bleeding.
- Organ damage.
- 'Failure' (drain requires repositioning or reinserting).
- Vasovagal reactions are not uncommon.
- Death related to either RPO or organ puncture.

Patients should give appropriate consent for the procedure and be informed of the complications.

Insertion technique

General preparation

- Obtain written consent.
- Confirm the side of the effusion at bedside via thoracic ultrasound.
- Ensure assistant available and drain bottle/tubing prepared.
- Choose drain insertion site:
  - Most chest drains are inserted at the fourth or fifth intercostal space in the anterior axillary or midaxillary line.
  - Aim for the 'triangle of safety' for majority of pneumothorax to avoid major vessels and nerves (an area posterior to pectoralis major, anterior to latissimus dorsi, and above the nipple line).
- Use real-time ultrasound to assess best position for drain insertion for pleural effusions—mark at the bedside.
- Possible positions include patient sitting upright and leaning forward with their arms raised and resting on a table in front of them or lying flat on their side in the fetal position to allow easy access to the safety triangle.
- Sterile technique: don gloves and gown; prepare skin by cleaning with chlorhexidine and drape area.
- Infiltrate with local anaesthetic as per pleural aspiration (1% lidocaine 10–20 ml may be required) and ensure pleural fluid (effusion) or air (pneumothorax) is aspirated easily using the 21G local anaesthetic needle.
- A longer needle (e.g. spinal needle) may be required in obese patients but proceed cautiously.
- If fluid/air is not easily aspirated, abandon procedure and request image guidance.

Seldinger drain insertion

After the steps above, proceed as follows.

- While waiting for local anaesthetic to take effect, open and prepare the Seldinger drain kit.
- Insert the introducer needle attached to the syringe (over the rib). Carefully advance the needle while aspirating. The introducer needles are not sharp and should be advanced in a controlled manner. Advance until fluid/air is easily aspirated; if you cannot aspirate easily you must abandon the procedure.
- Detach syringe and thread guidewire through introducer needle. The guidewire should pass without resistance.
- From this point, one hand must always be holding the guidewire. Remove the introducer needle over the wire.
- Make a small 1 cm incision in the skin around the guidewire with the scalpel.
- Thread the dilator over the guidewire and insert 2–3 cm into the patient (no further). Withdraw the dilator over the wire. For larger chest drains there will be multiple dilators; pass these sequentially to dilate the tract.
- Thread the drain over the guidewire until the wire emerges from the distal end of the drain. Insert the drain smoothly into the pleural space whilst holding on to the guidewire. Insertion to 10–14 cm is usually adequate.

- Remove guidewire (+ plastic drain stiffener) and attach three-way tap.
- Secure the chest drain with holding suture (a closing suture is not required) and commercial tube holder (usually part of chest drain kit). Cover with adhesive dressings.
- Connect to chest drain tubing and bottle. Bottles need to be primed with water up to the fill line. Ensure that:
  - drain is swinging
  - pleural fluid is draining (effusion) OR
  - drain is bubbling (pneumothorax).
- Ensure that the patient is aware of good drain care (e.g. do not lift above waist height).
- Request CXR to confirm position.
- Document procedure in medical notes, including any complications/ difficulties with drain insertion.

Blunt dissection insertion (trocar/Portex)

After general preparation:

- Make a 2–3 cm skin incision parallel to the ribs using a scalpel.
- Place a horizontal mattress suture across the wound using strong suture material (e.g. 1 silk).
- Create a tract for drain entry by blunt dissection using blunt forceps (e.g. Spencer–Wells) as follows.
  - Insert forceps (closed) into the incision and exert gentle pressure on the underlying tissue.
  - Open the forceps (separates underlying tissue).
  - Withdraw forceps completely while open.
  - Reinsert closed forceps and repeat steps above.
- The forceps should never be withdrawn in the closed position. This risks avulsion and damage to tissues.
- A 'give' will be felt on penetrating the parietal pleura. This may take some time, but attempting to rush blunt dissection can result in injury.
- Insert a finger through the tract into the pleural space to confirm correct position and to make sure there are no adhesions between lung and pleural surface.
- Clamp the chest drain tube at the insertion end with the clamp. With the aid of the clam insert the chest drain through the tract into the pleural space. Direct the chest drain either apically for a pneumothorax or inferiorly for pleural effusion. The drain should pass easily with minimal pressure.
- If there is resistance to passing the drain, **do not** exert firmer pressure (risks penetrating injury). Instead, repeat blunt dissection to re-create a tract and then attempt to re-pass the drain.
- Hold the drain in place, insert a holding suture.
- Continue management as per Seldinger drain insertion.

Part 6

Investigations

Chapter 50

Arterial blood gases

Introduction

Arterial blood gas (ABG) analysis forms the cornerstone of emergency respiratory investigation. In many situations values obtained dictate management strategy and facilitate decision making. It is an uncomfortable procedure for the patients and if repeated ABGs are required, consider whether less invasive measures, such as respiratory rate, pulse oximetry, or capillary blood gas measurements could be used.

Prior to every ABG—decide how the result will CHANGE MANAGEMENT

Principles

Technique and analysis

- Radial artery most commonly punctured. Alternative sites include femoral, ulnar, or brachial arteries.
- Capillary ear lobe samples can be used but can be difficult to obtain in an emergency setting.
- Introduction of a small superficial bleb of 1% lidocaine has been shown to significantly reduce levels of patient discomfort.
- If frequent gases are needed (e.g. commencing non-invasive ventilation) consider placement of an arterial line (see next page).
- Transport on ice is unnecessary if time to analysis is less than 10 minutes.
- Pre-analytical errors should be kept to minimum—see below.
- Analysis after change in therapy depends upon alveolar ventilation. 5 minutes is sufficient in most cases, however in obstructive airways disease steady state change may take up to 30 minutes.
- Always record the current FiO_2 and level of ventilatory support (as relevant).

The analyser

- **Beware** some values are measured (PaO_2, $PaCO_2$, pH) and others are 'calculated' (HCO_3, TCO, base excess, and often SaO_2—unless co-oximeter—see Chapter 51 'Pulse oximetry'). Calculated values are obtained from standardised equations that may not be appropriate or indeed accurate in critically ill patients.
- It is not uncommon for a busy machine to become decalibrated (e.g. over a bank holiday weekend) and therefore interpret unexpected results with caution.

ABG analytical errors

- **Too much heparin:** Liquid heparin must be expelled prior to sample collection (a small amount will always remain). The PaO_2 and $PaCO_2$ of heparin is virtually the same as ambient air and therefore heparin dilution will move the PaO_2 towards atmospheric values and (because it is acidic) lower the pH. Dry heparin syringes reduce this risk and allow for more accurate electrolyte calculation.
- **Exposed to air:** Sample will tend toward ambient room values. $PaCO_2$ reduced, pH increased.
- **Slow analysis:** aside from exposure to air, blood continues to metabolise and hence the PaO_2 decreases, $PaCO_2$ increases, and pH falls.
- **? *Venous:*** is often seen scrawled next to ABG printouts. Pulsatile flow may be poor in the critically ill patient. Compare SaO_2 with pulse oximeter—usually fairly good correlation, however, if there is still clinically significant doubt analyse a venous sample.
- **Temperature correction?** Most blood gas analysers maintain the electrode at 37°C. If the patient is relatively hypothermic, the electrode will heat the sample and reduce the Hb affinity, raising the PaO_2 (the reverse is also true). Most analysers incorporate equations to adjust for this effect (and hence change all calculated values). Changes in acid base status may reflect in vivo homeostasis and therefore should be interpreted according to unadjusted values.

When to consider an arterial line in respiratory emergencies

- In the **critically ill patient** who is likely to need close blood pressure monitoring (e.g. in setting of inotrope use, haemodynamically unstable).

Those likely to **need multiple ABGs**. Patients on non-invasive ventilation often fall into this group however consider other variables that can be used to assess progress; transcutaneous CO_2 monitoring has been shown to be useful.

When placing a line consider

- Remember Allen's Test prior to insertion (testing patency of ulnar and radial arterial flow)—demonstrated at weblink below.
- Ensure every sample taken has implications for management.
- Venesection of patient if multiple samples taken (including wastage for clearing line)—watch for falling Hb.
- Remove at first opportunity—infectious risk lower than venous access but remains source of sepsis.

Technique is demonstrated in the video at the following link: http://content.nejm.org/cgi/video/354/15/e13/
DOI:10.1056/NEJMvcm044149

Simple questions for ABG interpretation

It is important to consider the following questions to optimise interpretation. They can be approached in any order:

1) Is the sample correctly analyzed?

Reduce analytic errors—See previous section.

2) What does the ABG tell you about oxygen delivery?

See Chapter 42 for more details but key is SaO_2, PaO_2, and Hb (if measured). Patients are often on high FiO_2 and therefore it is important to always record and consider the FiO_2. E.g. PaO_2 14 on FiO_2 0.6 (60 %) is not good!

Quick check

Is the PaO_2 as high as expected?

If the $PaCO_2$ is normal, then the $PaCO_2$ (kPa) approximately = FiO_2 (%) × 0.75
e.g. as above 60 × 0.75 = 45 kPa

In addition to conditions that cause V/Q mismatch or shunting, a low PaO_2 may also arise due to hypoventilation—therefore one needs to calculate the A–a gradient (see below).

3) What is the $PaCO_2$?

$PaCO_2$ will give clues regarding ventilation—less than 4.0 kPa suggests hyperventilation, greater than 6.0 kPa suggests hypoventilation. It is important to remember that 'hypoventilation' may reflect an imbalance between load and capacity and not simply a low RR.

4) What is the pH?

If an acid base disturbance is present, determine the nature of the disturbance (see below). Beware compensation and look at base excess and HCO_3; significant disturbances may underlie a near normal pH.

5) What other information can help?

Look at all the information—view and record Mg, lactate, and COHb (is the patient still smoking?).

The alveolar to arterial gradient made simple

The A–a gradient is a measure of how efficiently the respiratory exchange surface is functioning. If the alveolus is packed with CO_2 then there is less O_2 to exchange and this is reflected in the PaO_2. Calculating the A–a gradient allows determination of oxygen exchange with respect to CO_2 and FiO_2.

Example: In a drowsy patient with an elevated $PaCO_2$ and low PaO_2 the A–a gradient helps determine if the poor saturations can be purely attributed to hypoventilation or if there is an underlying abnormality of oxygen exchange, e.g. pulmonary embolus.

How is it calculated?

$$\text{A}-\text{a gradient} = \text{Alveolar PO}_2 - (\text{PaO}_2 + \text{PaCO}_2/\text{R})$$

The alveolar oxygen needs to be adjusted according to the FiO_2, atmospheric pressure (100 kPa) and water vapour pressure (7 kPa) as follows:

$$\text{FiO}_2\ \text{Air},\ 21/100 \times (100-7)\ \text{approx. 20 kPa}$$

$$\text{FiO}_2\ 24\%,\ 24/100 \times \left(100-7\right)\ \text{approx. 23 kPa}$$

$$\text{FiO}_2\ 35\%,\ 35/100 \times (100-7)\ \text{approx. 33 kPa}$$

Respiratory quotient (R) for purposes of on-call calculation = 0.8 (easier to multiply by 1.2).

Example

e.g. If breathing air (FiO_2 = 21 kPa), PaO_2 = 13 kPa and $PaCO_2$ = 4.8 kPa

Then the alveolar oxygen is 20

A–a gradient = 20 − (13+4.8/0.8) = 1

What is normal?

It is normal to have a small A–a gradient as, even in the normal lung, there is not perfect ventilation to perfusion matching. Values increase with age and are usually 1–2, increasing to 2–3 in the elderly.

Acid Base balance, pH, and respiratory emergencies

Key to acid base analysis is remembering that homeostasis is centred on maintaining near-normal pH; compensations are made to correct towards normal pH.

Larger texts describe in detail the nature of acid base abnormalities and compensatory mechanisms (see the *Oxford Handbook of Respiratory Medicine*, Appendix 1) however the most commonly encountered derangements in respiratory emergencies are:

Respiratory acidosis

1° *disturbance*: inadequate ventilation (best thought of as an imbalance between load on the system versus capacity) leading to elevated CO_2 and hence acidosis, e.g. neuromuscular respiratory failure.

Compensatory mechanism: retain HCO_3. Note some HCO_3 elevation occurs by virtue of acute buffering (haemoglobin and proteins). It is very unusual for full compensation to occur—therefore the primary disturbance can usually be deduced (although not in mixed pattern). Compensation occurs over a number of hours/days and hence pH and HCO_3 provide clues to the chronicity of a respiratory acidosis.

Respiratory alkalosis

1° *disturbance*: 'over' ventilation with low $PaCO_2$. E.g. hyperventilation. Can also occur in pathological conditions, e.g. pulmonary embolism and asthma.

Compensatory mechanism: waste HCO_3 leading to negative base excess. This can give clues to 'chronicity' of dyspnoea.

Metabolic acidosis

1° *disturbance*: metabolic acid excess. In emergencies think about lactate, renal function, glucose, drugs, toxins, and alcohol. If still unclear then determine anion gap (normal range = 8–16 mmol/L).

$$\text{Anion gap} = [K^+] + [Na^+] - [Cl^-] - [HCO_3^-]$$

Tissue hypoxia leads to anaerobic metabolism and hence lactate production.

Large doses of salbutamol can give rise to lactic acidosis.

Metabolic acidosis and ↑ anion gap

Due to increased production of fixed/organic acids:

- Lactic acidosis—shock, infection, hypoxia.
- Renal failure.
- DKA (and ketone production in alcohol excess).
- Drugs/toxins (salicylates, biguanides, ethylene glycol, methanol).

Metabolic acidosis and normal anion gap

Due to loss of bicarbonate or ingestion of H+ ions:

- Renal tubular acidosis.
- Diarrhoea.
- Drugs (acetazolamide).
- Addison's disease.
- Pancreatic fistula.

Compensatory mechanism: increased ventilatory drive with reduced $PaCO_2$—occurs acutely. May explain why the acidotic patient appears breathless and underpins why respiratory rate is such a sensitive marker for detecting the acutely unwell medical patient (as part of emergency warning scores).

Tips for acid base interpretation

- A falling pH in a patient with respiratory failure may occur secondary to a change in the metabolic component, e.g. secondary to lactic acidaemia. **Beware attributing falling pH to ventilatory deterioration.**
- pH is key to acute management decisions in ventilatory failure—see ➲ Chapter 44. In decompensation an approximate correction can be made for the pH to estimate where the 'chronic' $PaCO_2$ normally 'sits':

For every increase in $PaCO_2$ of 2.6 kPa above normal the pH falls by 0.1.
For every decrease of $PaCO_2$ of 1.3 kPa below normal the pH rises by 0.1.
Although this relationship is not entirely linear it can be used as a useful trick.

e.g. *in decompensated acute on chronic respiratory failure if the pH is 7.25 and the $PaCO_2$ 9.0, (providing the pH disturbance is predominantly respiratory), one would expect a $PaCO_2$ at 'compensation' (i.e. above 7.35) to be 9.0–2.6 -6.4.*

Other methods for assessing CO_2

Transcutaneous CO_2

$PaCO_2$ can be monitored using trans-cutaneous skin monitors. These have been previously used successfully in sleep laboratories but can be used to manage patients on NIV. Limitations include cost, risk of thermal skin burns, and skill requirement (poor care can lead to sensor damage).

End tidal CO_2

On call general physicians will most commonly encounter this technique when it is employed to monitor intubated patients. The technique utilises the principles of absorption spectroscopy to measure CO_2 in expired gas. It is most useful for detecting ET tube displacement (gastric trace obtained) and when transferring critically ill patients.

Pulse oximetry

Introduction

When employed correctly, pulse oximetry is a rapid non-invasive method of assessing one of the key components of tissue oxygen delivery: the oxygen saturation of haemoglobin (SaO_2).

Principles and application

- Based on the laws of light absorbance and optical density (Lambert's law and Beer's law), i.e. the principle that deoxygenated and oxygenated haemoglobin absorb light at different wavelengths.
- The accuracy of modern pulse oximeters is ± 2%, although they are less accurate in lower saturation ranges. When inaccuracies occur saturation is usually underestimated. However, this underlines the need for **caution when reliance is placed on an absolute figure**, i.e. as a screening tool to avoid arterial blood gas sampling.
- A number of factors can affect accuracy and cause problems (see box 'Problems with pulse oximetry').

Pulse oximetry versus co-oximetry

- Pulse oximeters measure oxygen saturation SpO_2. This differs from the arterial saturation value (SaO_2) obtained in blood gas analysers with a CO-oximeter. In the latter, a larger number of wavelengths allow the measurement of other haemoglobin types:

$$SaO_2 = HbO_2 / (HbO_2 + Hb + COHb + metHb) \times 100\%$$

- In clinical practice the terms SpO_2 and SaO_2 are often used interchangeably. In the majority of circumstances this is of no consequence. However, it is important to understand that there is a difference.
- ⓘ **Beware** some analysers are not CO-oximeters and simply determine SaO_2 for wavelengths as per a finger probe.
- Co-oximetry is necessary in the management of carbon monoxide (CO) poisoning. COHb has similar absorbance and therefore mimics the presence of oxyhaemoglobin. This leads to falsely elevated SaO_2 readings on a standard saturation monitor.
- Smoking can also increase CO levels (often used in smoking cessation clinics as a tool to assess compliance) and can lead to SaO_2 inaccuracy (falsely elevated).

Other uses

- Overnight oximetry can be used to assess nocturnal desaturation in sleep-disorder breathing.

Problems with pulse oximetry

Common

- Signal quality: often due to probe application. Can try tape to secure probe or earlobe device.
- Tissue perfusion, e.g. hypotension.
- Body temperature.
- Penumbra: light shunting around the finger gives falsely low SaO_2.

Uncommon

- Nail varnish: effect depends upon colour. Green and blue reduce SaO_2 reading, but red usually has no effect. Aim to remove all varnish to obtain optimum reading.
- Anaemia (Hb <5).

Rare (low SaO_2 with no apparent explanation)

- Dyshaemoglobinaemia (see CO-oximeter entry above), e.g. methaemoglobinaemia. The wavelength light absorption leads SaO_2 towards 85%.
- Intravascular dyes.

Chapter 52

Peak flow

Introduction

Peak flow is defined as the greatest expiratory flow achieved from a maximally forced expiratory effort when starting from a position of full inspiration. It has the most clinical value in asthma.

Principles and application

- Measurement should be performed as best of three with standardised metre (EU scale). There is no need to return the measuring plunger to zero following each attempt.
- Result is effort-dependent.
- Circadian changes are well recognised: peaks at 16.00, nadir at 04.00.
- Guidelines suggest cut-off values to determine severity of acute asthma and dictate treatment. However, trends and response to treatment are more useful than absolute values. For reference range see Fig. 52.1.
- PEFR is affected by changes in large airway calibre and therefore is of limited value in the assessment of COPD.
- PEFR has no value in discriminating restrictive from obstructive disease: restrictive conditions will limit ability to generate high PEFR.

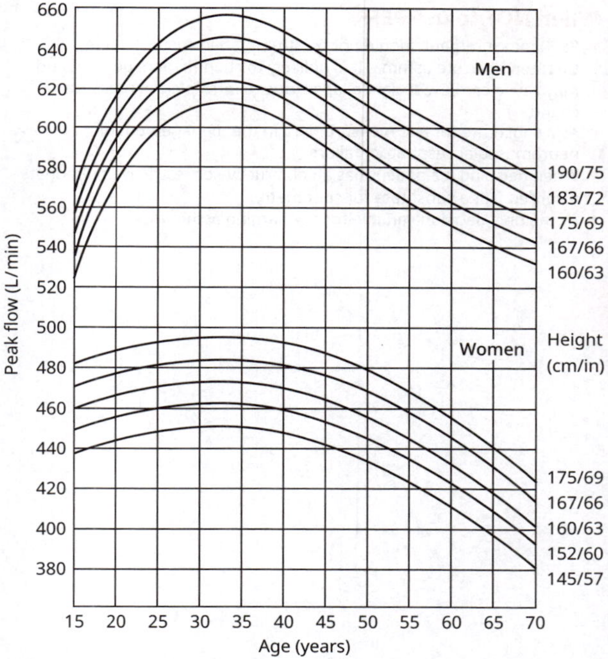

Fig. 52.1 Peak flow reference ranges. (With kind permission from Oxford University Press in *The Oxford Handbook of Respiratory Medicine*.)

When NOT to use PEFR

- PEFR measurement should not be attempted in suspected life-threatening acute asthma. It is unlikely to change management and may cause cardiovascular collapse (due to intra-pleural pressure changes).
- As a substitute for FVC measurement in the management of neuromuscular respiratory failure.
- When deciding if a patient has an obstructive or restrictive pulmonary disorder. Not a substitute for spirometry.
- As the only decision variable for discharging asthmatics.

Cough peak flow

Peak expiratory flow during cough (cough PEF) is a useful adjunct in the assessment of patients with suspected neuromuscular respiratory failure. Values below 150 L/min suggest poor airway clearance and should prompt consideration of further investigation and intervention to ensure adequate management.

Chapter 53

Spirometry

Introduction

When performed correctly, spirometry is a valuable tool which helps to classify a respiratory disorder. It is rarely indicated in the acute emergency setting, although is of significant importance in the management of patients with neuromuscular respiratory failure (FVC monitoring).

Principles

- Modern hand-held electronic devices allow simple analysis.
- Effort- and technique-dependent. The patient breathes at tidal volume, then inhales slowly to total lung capacity (TLC), and then exhales as hard and fast as possible to residual volume (RV). Encouragement should be given to ensure maximum force and continuation. It is important to use a spirometer with a volume–time trace to ensure that the true FVC is obtained.
- Repeatability is the key to ensuring that adequate patient effort has been obtained.
- Many devices enable calculation of a predicted value (for age, sex, and height). If they do not, good calculators are available at: http://www.cdc.gov/niosh/topics/spirometry/RefCalculator.html
- When interpreting values, 'normal' is usually taken to include values >80% of the predicted value. However, it is perhaps more useful to consider predicted values in terms of a range around the population mean ± 1.64 × standard deviation.
- It is important to consider the population data you are using. There are no accurate population data for people aged >85 years.
- Do not confuse the results for the FEV_1/FVC ratio (FER) and the percentage predicted figure with that ratio sometimes given on electronic printouts. Use the actual percentage (in bold below). For example:

$FEV_1 = 1.94$, FVC = 2.60, age 50 years, height 1.60 m

FEV_1 / FVC = 74%

Percentage predicted 90%

Spirometry application

- Most commonly used to distinguish restrictive from obstructive disorders. FEV_1/FVC <0.7 is suggestive of the latter (see Table 53.1).
- In restrictive disorders the ratio is usually preserved due to fall in FVC. ❗ Beware. Not all falls in FVC are due to restrictive disease. FVC also falls if RV is elevated (due to air trapping) (see Fig. 53.1).
- Percentage predicted values for FEV_1 help to classify severity of disease in COPD and guide treatment (➲ Chapter 21). FEV_1 does not change significantly during exacerbations and is of limited value in monitoring.

Table 53.1 Pattern of lung volume change found in obstructive and restrictive lung disease

Derivative	Obstructive	Restrictive
FEV_1 (% predicted)	↓↓	↓
VC (% predicted)	↓ or →	↓
FEV_1/VC ratio	↓	→ or ↑ (increased recoil)
TLC (% predicted)	↑ orl	↓
RV (% predicted)	↑	↓
FRC (% predicted)	↑	↓
RV/TLC ratio	↑ (gas trapping)	↓ *

Reproduced from the *Oxford Handbook of Respiratory Medicine* with permission from Oxford University Press.

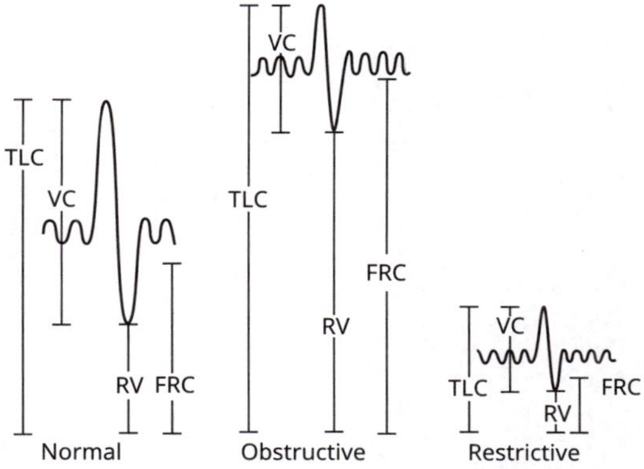

Fig. 53.1 Lung volumes in normal, obstructive, and restrictive lung conditions.

Abbreviations: FEV_1, forced expiratory volume in 1 second; FRC, functional residual capacity; RV, residual volume; TLC, total lung capacity; VC, vital capacity.

Reproduced from the *Oxford Handbook of Respiratory Medicine* with kind permission from Oxford University Press.

- FVC monitoring in neuromuscular respiratory failure: if the diaphragm is paralysed then on lying flat the abdominal contents limit inspiration. Early failure may be detected by supine drop in FVC:
- 10–20 % is suspicious; >20% is definitely abnormal and suggests significance, usually bilateral paralysis. (Note: Drops by 5% in normal subjects.) Do not substitute PEFR for FVC in this condition.

For more details see the *Oxford Handbook of Respiratory Medicine*, Appendix 6.

Further pulmonary function tests

A number of other pulmonary function tests are widely available and used in respiratory medicine (e.g. formal lung function tests/body plethysmography, transfer factor analysis). However, in the **emergency setting** it is probably more important to ask the following questions:

- Will the investigation I am requesting change management acutely?
- Can the patient safely undergo the investigation and perform sufficiently to achieve a meaningful result?
- Do I know what the 'normal' values should be and how a certain result is interpreted?

For example, in the setting of suspected acute pulmonary haemorrhage requesting transfer factor analysis. Visit the pulmonary function technicians and discuss what is feasible and sensible. Novel techniques may be available (such as using trans-diaphragmatic pressure recordings), but again ask local specialist/technicians for advice.

The Empey index

The Empey index is a method of predicting whether a patient has upper airways obstruction:

$$\text{Empey index} = FEV_1/PEFR$$

In the presence of upper airways obstruction PEFR is reduced disproportionately to FEV_1. A figure >10 supports the presence of upper airways obstruction. The index has been used at the bedside to support a diagnosis of tracheal stenosis.

Chapter 54

Bronchoscopy

Introduction

Bronchoscopy involves the passage of a fibreoptic bronchoscope through the upper airways, past the vocal cords, and into the lungs. The upper and lower airways can be examined, samples can be taken for diagnosis, and treatment can be carried out if necessary. There are only a few indications for urgent bronchoscopy, which are discussed below. The opinion of a respiratory physician should be sought.

Indications for urgent bronchoscopy

Foreign body

Usually associated with a clear history of aspiration. CXR may show the foreign body if radio-opaque, or may show an area of atelectasis or hyperinflation on a post-expiration film. It is better seen on CT chest. The most common site for aspiration is the right lower lobe. Bronchoscopy is only required urgently if there is respiratory distress.

Thoracic trauma

Bronchoscopy might be required to exclude serious airway injury such as tracheobronchial fracture. May also reveal aspirated foreign bodies or be useful therapeutically for removal of mucous plugs.

Massive haemoptysis

Occasionally indicated in massive haemoptysis. Can be a useful test to localise the site of bleeding. If bleeding is localised to a distal bronchus, attempt to tamponade by wedging the bronchoscope into the bronchus. Iced saline can be irrigated or use 1 ml aliquots of 1:10 000 adrenaline onto the bleeding point to arrest the bleeding. If available, attempt to coagulate the bleeding point. Uncontrollable bleeding ideally requires a rigid bronchoscope, usually only done by thoracic surgeons.

Causes include neoplasm, tuberculous cavities, aspergillomas, pulmonary alveolar haemorrhage syndromes, bronchiectasis, and cystic fibrosis. Death occurs secondary to asphyxiation not exsanguination. If there is massive bleeding turn patient onto the side of the bleeding to protect the other lung. Consider intubation with double lumen tube (➲ Chapter 6)

Usual indications for bronchoscopy

- Suspected lung cancer, for staging and histology or cytology.
- Suspected mycobacterial disease, where the patient is unable to produce sputum.
- In the immunocompromised patient with fever/hypoxia/pulmonary infiltrates and negative sputum samples (➲ Chapter 13).
- Diffuse interstitial lung disease: transbronchial biopsy is performed rarely now but can be used to obtain histology. Often positive in sarcoidosis but less helpful in other conditions.
- For therapeutic intervention, e.g. stenting, diathermy.

Contraindications

- Unstable cardiovascular state, including arrhythmias.
- Severe hypoxaemia that is likely to worsen during the procedure.
- Uncooperative patient.
- Rigid bronchoscopy is contraindicated in those with severe ankylosing spondylitis of the neck or in the presence of an unstable cervical spine.

Preparation pre-bronchoscopy

- Full history including allergies and previous response to anaesthetic.
- Examination of cardiovascular and respiratory systems.
- CXR.
- Clotting screen and platelet count if intervention procedures likely or if on anticoagulants or concerns re. clotting status (e.g. liver metastases, uraemia).
- Fast for 4 hours pre-procedure.
- Consent.

Other considerations pre-bronchoscopy

- If the patient has asthma, consider pre-bronchoscopy nebuliser of short-acting beta-agonist.
- Because of the requirement to be nil by mouth pre-bronchoscopy, consideration must be given to diabetics' medication.
- Patients with potential transmissible organisms should be performed at the end of the list.

Complications

Mortality and morbidity are low with bronchoscopy. However, complications can arise related to the use of sedation, topical anaesthetics, or the procedure itself.

Complications from sedation include respiratory depression, syncope, and hypotension. Rarely, topical anaesthetics may cause laryngospasm or bronchospasm. Cardiac arrhythmias occur in ~0.5%. Haemorrhage associated with biopsy is one of the major complications and should be treated as discussed earlier in the chapter. Death related to bronchoscopy is extremely rare, occurring in <0.04%.

Patient post-bronchoscopy

Up to one-third of patients will develop fever after bronchoscopy and lavage (induced by cytokine release from alveolar macrophages). This will settle without antibiotics, although antipyretics such as paracetamol can be used.

In patients who have undergone interventional bronchoscopy such as diathermy or stenting, fever post-bronchoscopy should be treated with antibiotics (e.g. co-amoxiclav or doxycycline) as it is more likely to be due to infection.

Major complications include the following.

- Post-biopsy haemorrhage: if small volume then likely to settle. Consider admission for observation, particularly if significant volumes. ➲ Chapter 6 for management.
- Pneumothorax: occurs in ~10% after transbronchial lung biopsy. Consider in those presenting with chest pain and/or increased shortness of breath. Perform CXR and treat as per secondary pneumothorax.

Chapter 55

Radiology

Introduction

Because of its portable nature and rapid interpretation, the posteroanterior (PA) chest X-ray (CXR) (Fig. 55.1) remains the most useful radiological investigation for the patient with acute respiratory symptoms. Accurate assessment of the CXR is based on a combination of pattern recognition and a logical approach to ensure that important features on the film are not missed or misinterpreted. The experienced physician will use the CXR to assess not only the lungs, but also the trachea, mediastinum, hila, pleura, bones, and chest wall.

In this chapter we describe the important CXR patterns for the most common respiratory emergencies. If another imaging modality is needed to confirm the diagnosis, the investigation of choice will be described.

Infection

The CXR appearances of infection are extremely varied. A bacterial infection causing community-acquired pneumonia (CAP) may be seen as a solitary focus of consolidation, whereas PCP in the immunocompromised patient typically causes a bilateral peri-hilar infiltrate. Whilst familiarity with the features of CAP on CXR will enable prompt treatment to be started, the physician must also recognise complications of infection, such as a lung abscess or cavitation. The indicative signs for an atypical, viral, or fungal infection must also be known.

CXR features of bacterial infection (Fig. 55.2)

- Consolidation (dense shadowing that obscures blood vessels), often with air bronchograms (visible airways within the shadowing).
- Lower lobes most commonly affected.
- Pleural effusion is common, but lymphadenopathy is uncommon.
- A more diffuse interstitial and infiltrative pattern can be seen without focal consolidation.
- Consolidation can appear as a discrete focal mass, mimicking or possibly obscuring an underlying malignancy. ! A repeat CXR 6 weeks after treatment is advised to exclude a lung cancer.
- Multifocal consolidation can be seen, particularly in streptococcal infection.

Other CXR features: consider atypical infection

- Unstable cardiovascular state cavitation (round lucency, often multifocal): seen especially with *Staphylococcus aureus* infection. Pneumothorax (PTX) can be a complication.
- Differential of cavitation on the CXR.
  - Infection: predominantly *staphylococcus*, but also anaerobes and fungal.
  - Tuberculosis (TB).
  - Carcinoma.
  - Granulomatous vasculitis.
  - Rheumatoid nodules.
- Upper lobe predilection: seen especially with *Klebsiella* and TB.
- Lower lobe predilection: seen especially with *Legionella*.

CXR features of viral pneumonia

- Bilateral diffuse infiltrate as opposed to focal consolidation.
- Multiple nodules,1–5 mm in diameter.
- Calcification of nodules implies prior, not active, infection (especially varicella).
- Effusions and hilar lymphadenopathy are not typically present.
- Bacterial infection can complicate viral pneumonia.

CXR features of fungal infection

Variable findings, but there is generally a diffuse infiltrative or nodular appearance. Some fungal infections have specific CXR features.

- Aspergilloma or mycetoma: usually an apical cavity containing a fungal ball of soft tissue density. Surrounding crescent of air visible (halo sign). A complication of cavitatory TB.
- Bronchopulmonary aspergillosis: CXR shows central bronchiectasis (airway dilatation). Mucoid impaction within these dilated airways gives a 'finger in glove' appearance.
- PCP: bilateral peri-hilar opacity. Occasionally small cysts may be seen. CXR normal in 10%. PTX a common complication. PCP should be considered in at-risk patients presenting with pneumothorax.

Tuberculosis

TB has perhaps the most variable appearance on CXR of any infection, sometimes complicated by prior surgical treatment. Certain CXR features should alert the clinician to the possibility of tuberculous disease, although comparison with old films is often necessary to assess whether CXR abnormalities are longstanding (Fig. 55.3).

CXR features suggestive of TB

- Upper lobe consolidation.
- Hilar or paratracheal lymph node enlargement. Main differential is sarcoid (Fig. 55.4).
- Cavitation (hallmark of reactivation), possibly with mycetoma.
- Multiple nodules 2–3 mm in size are characteristic of miliary TB (diffuse haematogenous spread).

Role of ultrasound and CT

An ultrasound scan (US) should be performed if an effusion or empyema is suspected and the CXR is not diagnostic. If a lung abscess is suspected, CT is highly sensitive and specific. Some lung abscesses are amenable to percutaneous drainage under CT guidance.

High-resolution CT scanning (HRCT) is the investigation of choice when fungal infection is suspected, especially for patients who are immunocompromised. Some organisms, particularly PCP and invasive aspergillosis, have characteristic appearances on HRCT, and this investigation can be diagnostic.

Pneumothorax

PTX is air in the pleural space, with consequent collapse of adjacent lung. The key CXR features are listed below. If a tension PTX is suspected and there are signs of imminent cardiovascular compromise, treatment should be undertaken before the CXR is performed.

CXR features of pneumothorax (Figs. 55.5 and 55.6)

- Abnormal lucency (blackness) within a hemithorax.
- Shift of trachea/mediastinum away from side of PTX (consider carefully whether tension PTX exists).
- A thin white line representing the visceral pleura may be seen, separating collapsed lung from air in the pleural space.
- Absence of vascular markings (although this is normal in the lung periphery).
- A ruptured pleural bleb may be seen in spontaneous PTX.
- Ipsilateral blunting of the costophrenic angle.
- Abnormal prominence and depth of the ipsilateral costophrenic angle (deep sulcus sign). Seen if patient has been imaged supine (e.g. ventilated patient on ITU).
- Medial diaphragm clearly outlined through cardiac silhouette or abnormal sharpness of a cardiac border, again usually seen in a supine patient with air lying anteriorly in the thorax.

Common pitfalls

- A rotated film can cause apparent lucency of one hemithorax (common when a portable CXR has been taken).
- Mistaking overlying clothing or even hair for the pleural edge.
- Bullae (in context of COPD) can mimic PTX as both cause abnormal lucency.

Further information

- Lateral decubitus or expiratory frontal CXR can reveal a small PTX not readily visible on the erect CXR.
- CT thorax is occasionally indicated in the context of gross bullous changes or presence of extensive surgical emphysema, making the CXR difficult to interpret.

Pulmonary embolism

Although there are no specific diagnostic CXR features, it should still be performed to exclude other pathologies.

Non-specific CXR features (often normal)

- Pleural effusion
- Small pleural effusion (usually exudate).
- Atelectasis (a focal area of collapse, usually linear or wedge-shaped).
- Decreased vascularity causing increased lucency of a lobe or hemithorax (Westermark sign).
- Prominence of a pulmonary artery.
- Raised hemidiaphragm.

Further investigations

CT pulmonary angiogram (CTPA)

- The investigation of choice with a sensitivity >95%.
- Requires 100 ml of IV contrast through a large-bore peripheral cannula.
- Contraindicated if the patient has renal failure, severe asthma, or a history of allergy to iodine.
- Acute emboli seen as low-attenuation filling defects in pulmonary vasculature.
- CTPA has the advantage of demonstrating other causes for respiratory symptoms in the absence of PE.

Isotope lung scan (ventilation/perfusion or V/Q scan)

- Ventilation and lung perfusion are studied by measuring the radioactivity of inhaled and injected particles. A perfusion defect in an area of normal ventilation is indicative of thrombus.
- Useful as a first-line investigation in patients with a normal CXR and no cardiac or pulmonary disease.
- Most commonly, only Q scan performed.
- Abnormal CXR often gives an indeterminate scan.
- CTPA preferred in most centres, although Q scan useful if CTPA is contraindicated and CXR is normal.

Out of hours availability

Many hospitals do not provide on-call nuclear medicine studies. CTPA can be delayed until normal working hours if there is no contraindication to anticoagulation in the interim.

Pleural effusion and empyema

Pleural effusion

Most effusions are easily seen on CXR and do not require further imaging. Ultrasound is required for further evaluation.

CXR features (Figs. 55.7 and 55.8)

- Basal opacity obscuring the hemidiaphragms.
- Meniscus curving upwards at the medial/lateral edges on the frontal view.
- Large effusions cause the mediastinum to be pushed away (cf. lobar collapse).
- Small effusions: only feature may be 'blunting' of the costophrenic angle.

Pitfalls

- Up to 200 ml of fluid can collect in the posterior recess and may not be seen on the PA CXR (a lateral CXR or US may be helpful).
- Fluid can also collect in the subpulmonic space, which is above the hemidiaphragm and inferior to the lung. The appearance is of an elevated hemidiaphragm, but with an abnormal lateral peak.

Empyema

This is infected pleural fluid and requires aspiration or drainage. The CXR cannot confirm or exclude whether pleural fluid is infected. US is useful for guiding percutaneous aspiration or chest drain insertion. This is especially true if the collection is small and/or loculated. If a patient with a chest infection remains septic despite treatment, a CT of the thorax will identify if an empyema or abscess is present.

CT features of empyema

- Low-attenuation collection between lung and the chest wall/mediastinum/diaphragm.
- Visceral and parietal pleura are separated.
- Pleura is thickened and shows avid enhancement with IV contrast.
- Foci of gas within the empyema (prior to pleural instrumentation) are suggestive of development of a bronchopleural fistula.

Pulmonary oedema and acute respiratory distress syndrome

There are many non-cardiac causes of pulmonary oedema and ARDS. These two pathologies are considered together as many of the CXR features overlap (the heart size and clinical presentation usually allow differentiation of the two). ARDS is common in ITU patients as a result of sepsis, aspiration, or DIC. Inhalation of smoke or overdose from opiate abuse are other causes. CXR features can lag behind the clinical status by 12–24 hours.

CXR features (Fig. 55.9)

- Prominence of upper lobe blood vessels ('upper lobe diversion').
- Peripheral horizontal linear shadows 1–2 cm long and 1 mm thick ('Kerley B lines').
- Pleural effusions (usually small and bilateral but can be large and unilateral).
- Peri-hilar shadowing ('batwing' shadowing). Implies acute severe oedema.
- Peri-bronchial cuffing (wall-thickening of large proximal airways).
- Multiple ill-defined nodules (air-space shadowing) seen bilaterally (late severe sign).
- Widespread consolidative pattern with air bronchograms. Can be indistinguishable from diffuse infection.
- Normal CTR seen in ARDS compared with increased CTR in pulmonary oedema.

Common pitfalls

Signs of pulmonary oedema are usually bilateral, but can be unilateral, e.g. ITU patient nursed on their side, unilateral aspiration or re-expansion pulmonary oedema after treatment of large pleural effusion.

Chronic obstructive pulmonary disease and asthma

The CXR of patients with chronic airway obstruction often displays features of lung hyperinflation with no focal abnormality.

CXR features of chronic airflow obstruction

- Lung hyperexpansion, causing flattening of the hemidiaphragms and increased lucency ('black lungs').
- Dome of diaphragm lies below anterior aspect of seventh rib.
- Abrupt tapering of the peripheral vasculature.
- Presence of bullae (much more common in COPD than in asthma). Basal predominance for bullae is highly suggestive of alpha-1-antitrypsin deficiency.
- Enlarged pulmonary arteries or right heart (as a result of chronic hypoxia).

If these background changes are observed, look for the common complications associated with COPD and asthma.

Complications

- PTX and surgical emphysema.
- Pneumomediastinum.
- Infection.
- Malignancy.
- Bronchiectasis (abnormally dilated airways which can contain fluid levels).
- Allergic bronchopulmonary aspergillosis.

Further imaging

Other imaging modalities are rarely needed in the acute setting. The main use of CT in the acute setting would be to identify a pneumothorax on a background of extensive bullous changes.

Massive haemopytsis

Life-threatening haemoptysis requires urgent resuscitation (➔ Chapter 1). The most common causes of massive haemoptysis and the associated CXR features are as follows.

CXR features

- Irregular focal mass: probably lung primary malignancy eroding an adjacent vessel.
- Consolidation: suggests infection. TB possible.
- Cavity and soft tissue mass: aspergilloma.
- Cavity with air–fluid level: lung abscess.
- Well-defined focal mass: arterio-venous malformation (AVM). Look for tubular feeding vessel. Multiple AVMs seen in Osler–Weber–Rendu syndrome.
- Dilated tubular bronchi or multiple cystic lucencies: bronchiectasis of any cause, but especially cystic fibrosis.

Further imaging may be required, usually CT of the thorax with contrast. A bronchial angiogram may be required when embolisation can also be performed as a therapeutic procedure. This needs to be performed at a specialist centre.

Lobar collapse

Lobar collapse (also known as 'atelectasis') is easy to miss on the frontal CXR unless it is specifically looked for. In the elderly patient an underlying malignancy is by far the most common cause, whereas an inhaled foreign body or mucus plug are more likely aetiologies in young patients. Whatever the cause, it is not a diagnosis that can be missed without consequence for the patient. Identifying the affected lobe will guide subsequent investigations, especially bronchoscopy.

General features of lobar collapse

- Opacification of the lobe.
- Displacement of the fissures (especially the horizontal).
- Volume loss on the affected side.
- Upward or downward shift of the hilum towards the collapsed lobe.
- Mediastinal shift towards the side of collapse.
- Poorly defined hemi-diaphragm/mediastinal contours (normally clearly seen).
- Elevation of the hemi-diaphragm.
- Rib crowding (best seen by comparing the gap between ribs on both sides).
- Hyperexpansion of the other lung, causing hyperlucency.
- Complete collapse of the entire lung causes opacification of the whole hemithorax, and ipsilateral shift of the mediastinum and trachea (Fig. 55.10).

Lobar specific features

Lobar collapse is one of the few indications for performing a lateral CXR if the frontal view is not confirmatory.

- RLL collapses posteriorly and inferiorly. Right hemi-diaphragm obscured.
- RML collapses anteriorly and medially, obscuring right heart border. Triangular opacity on lateral CXR.
- RUL collapses medially and superiorly.
- LUL (Fig. 55.11) Moves anteriorly and superiorly, creating a 'veil-like' appearance of the left hemi-thorax. Left heart border obscured. A crescent of aerated lung is often seen between the aortic arch and collapsed LUL (hyperexpanded apical segment of LLL).
- LLL (Fig. 55.12) The easiest lobar collapse to miss. Collapses posteriorly and inferiorly. Left hemidiaphragm obscured. Can appear as a triangular density behind the heart (the 'sail' sign). Often seen after cardiac surgery.

Further imaging

Post-IV contrast CT of the thorax is the next investigation, before bronchoscopy.

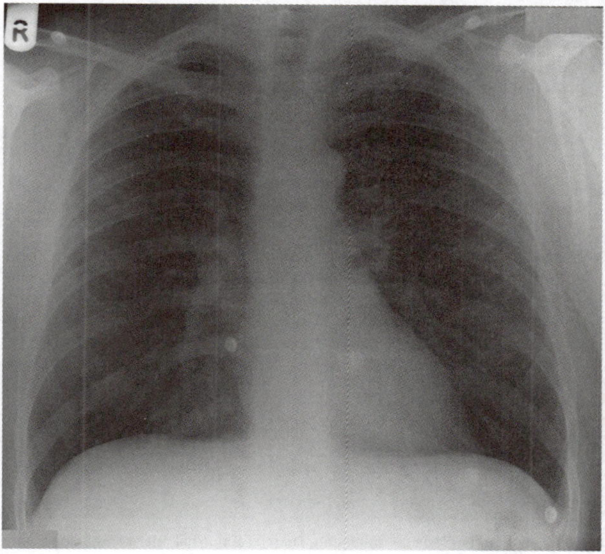

Fig. 55.1 Normal CXR. The heart size is normal and there are no focal lung lesions. Note how the heart borders and hemi-diaphragms are clearly visible.

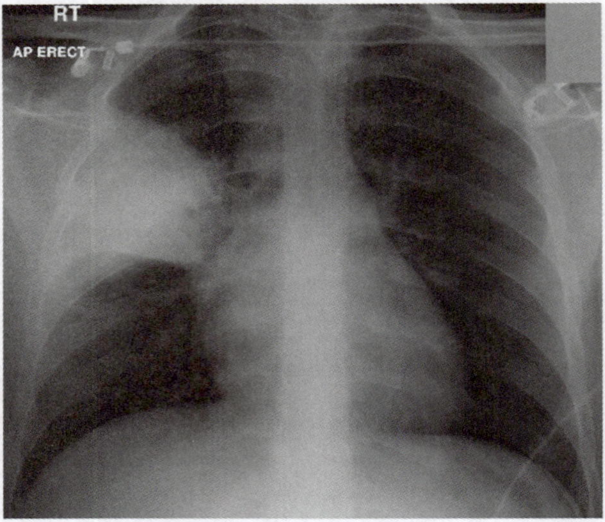

Fig. 55.2 Right upper lobe consolidation. There is abnormal opacity outlining a lung segment. An air bronchogram is seen adjacent to the right hilum.

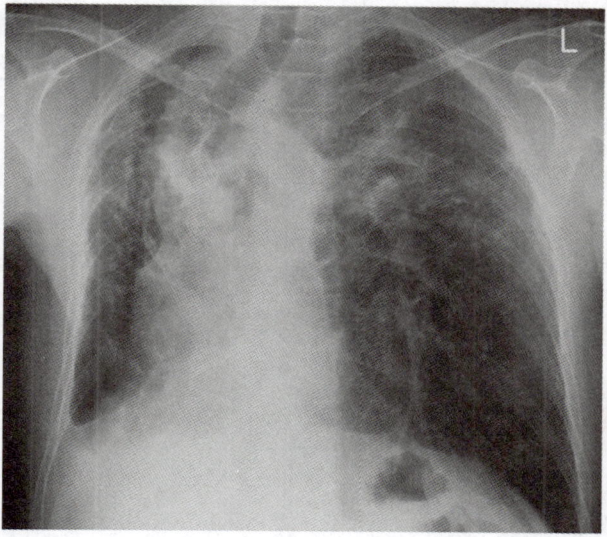

Fig. 55.3 Upper lobe fibrosis. Previous TB infection has caused extensive fibrotic change in the right upper lobe, with volume loss (note the elevated right hilum and tracheal shift), on a background of diffuse reticulonodular shadowing.

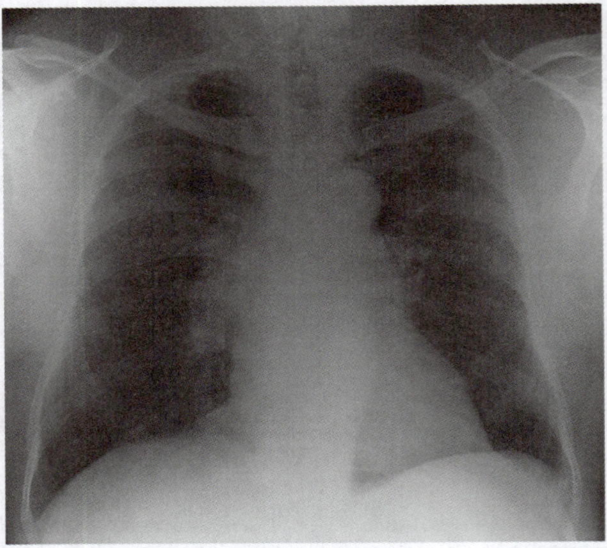

Fig. 55.4 Bilateral hilar lymphadenopathy. The hila are abnormally large and dense in this patient with sarcoid (compare with normal appearance in **Fig. 55.1**).

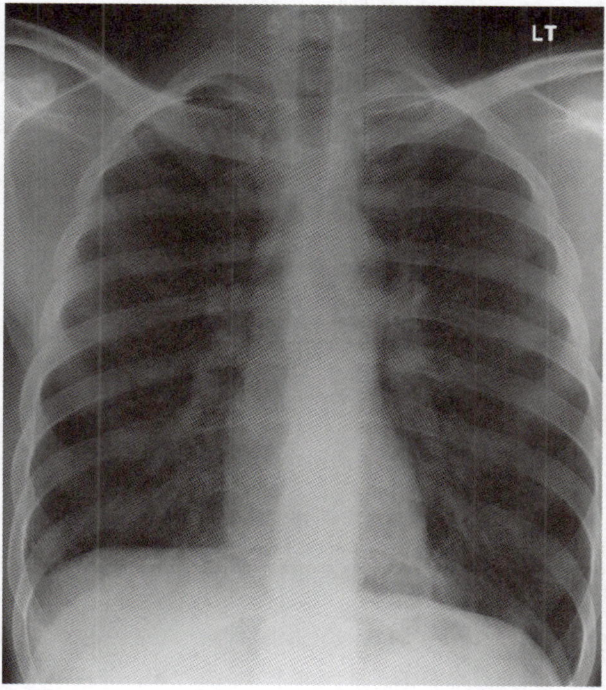

Fig. 55.5 Small pneumothorax. Abnormal lucency is seen parallel to the lateral chest wall, and a thin vertical line is present (representing the pleural edge). No mediastinal shift has occurred.

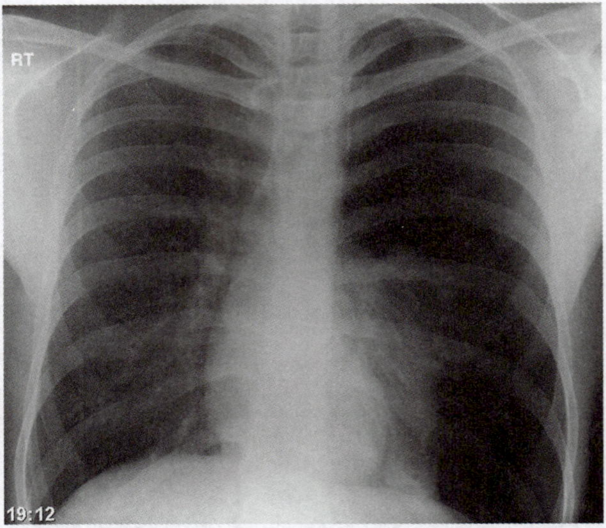

Fig. 55.6 Tension pneumothorax. There is complete collapse of the left lung, extensive air in the left pleural space, and mediastinal shift to the right.

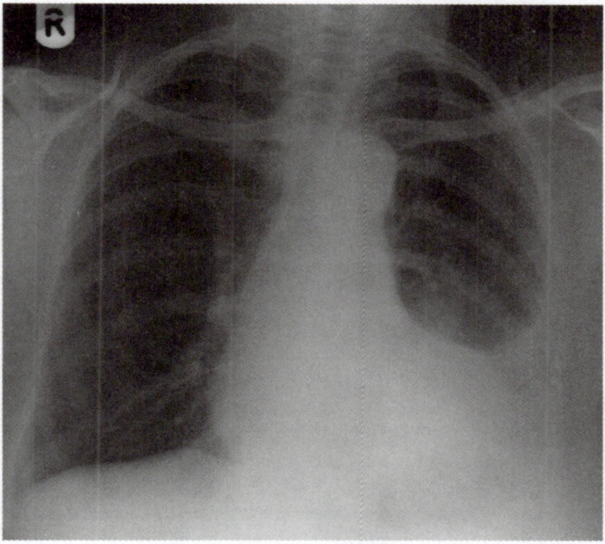

Fig. 55.7 Pleural effusion. Pleural fluid in the left pleural space is seen as abnormal opacity, with a meniscus extending along the lateral chest wall.

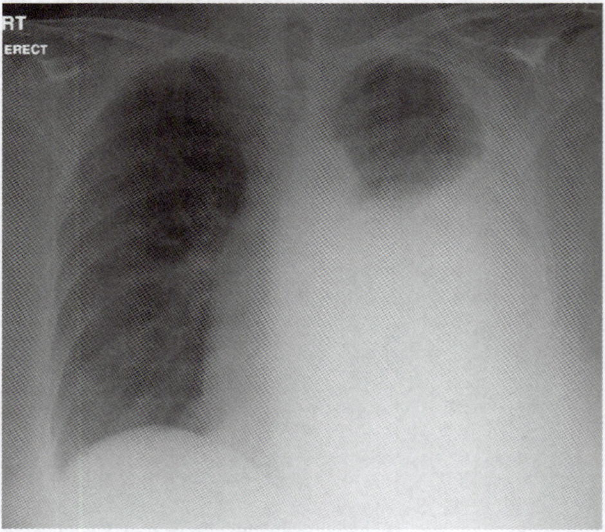

Fig. 55.8 Large pleural effusion. Extensive left-sided pleural fluid, causing shift of the trachea and mediastinum to the right.

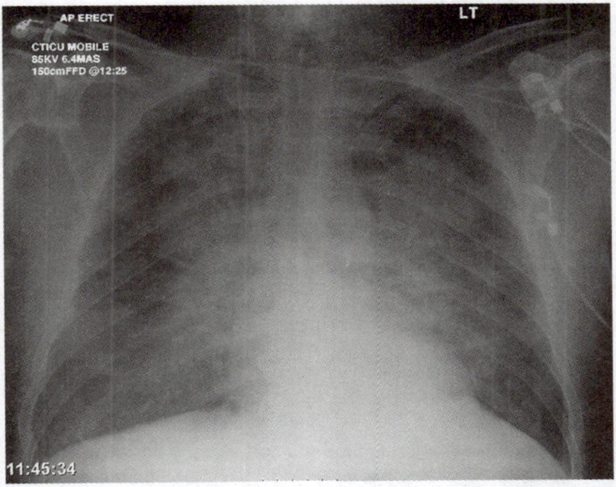

Fig. 55.9 Severe pulmonary oedema. 'Batwing', or peri-hilar air-space shadowing. Thin horizontal interstitial lines are seen laterally at the right base (Kerley B lines).

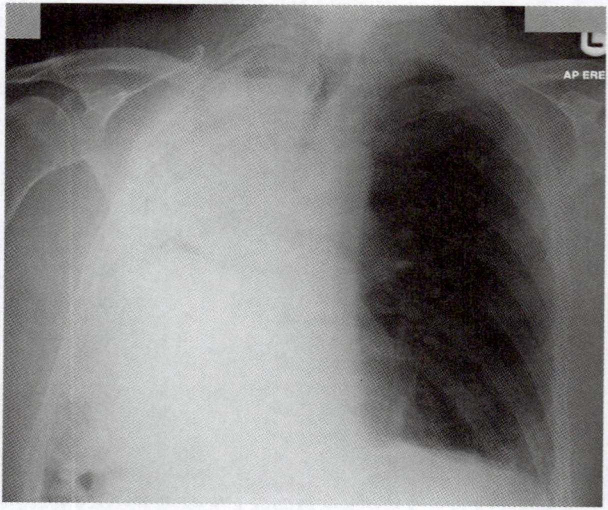

Fig. 55.10 Complete collapse of right lung. A proximal tumour is causing complete collapse of the right lung, seen as a 'white-out' with the trachea shifted towards the side of collapse (compare with a large pleural effusion which will shift the mediastinum away).

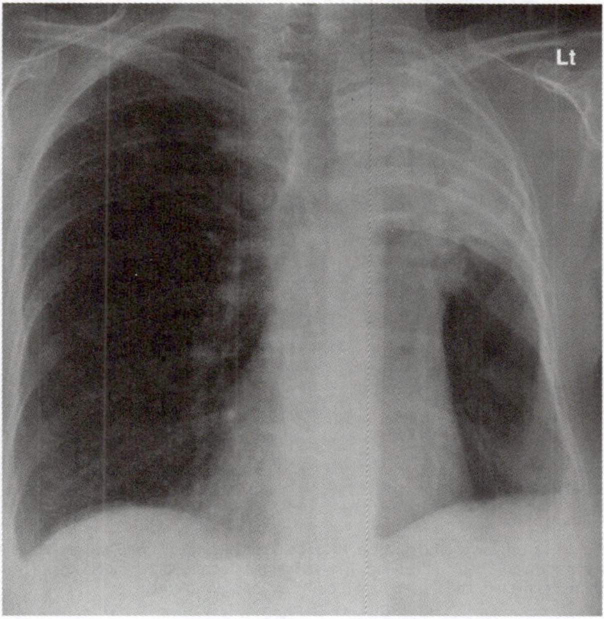

Fig. 55.11 Left upper lobe collapse. There is a mediastinal shift to the left, the left hilum is elevated, and there is abnormal density in the left upper zone. There is marked volume loss in the left hemithorax.

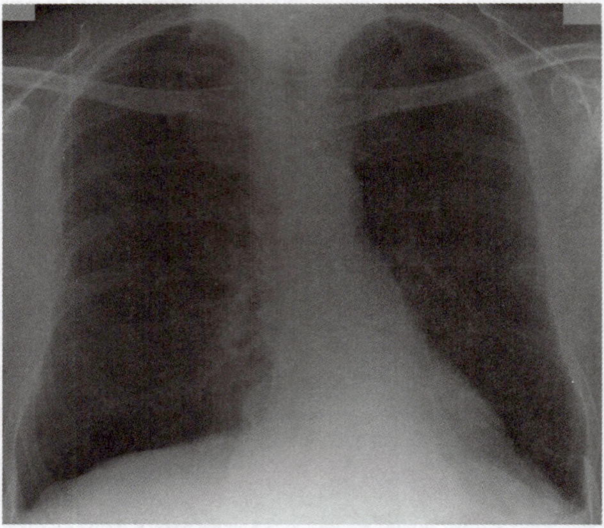

Fig. 55.12 Left lower lobe collapse. The lobe is completely collapsed and is seen as a dense triangle behind the heart. The left hilum is depressed, the mediastinum has shifted to the left, and the left hemithorax is of reduced volume.

Index

For the benefit of digital users, indexed terms that span two pages (e.g., 52–53) may, on occasion, appear on only one of those pages.

Tables, and figures are indicated by an italic *t*, and *f* following the page number.

A

B

C

D

Q

R

U

V

W

Z